Spiritual Care in Everyday Nursing Practice

Spiritual Care in Everyday Nursing Practice

A New Approach

Janice Clarke, RGN, PhD

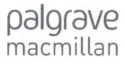

First published 2013 by
PALGRAVE MACMILLAN

Palgrave Macmillan in the UK is an imprint of Macmillan Publishers Limited, registered in England, company number 785998, of Houndmills, Basingstoke, Hampshire RG21 6XS.

Palgrave Macmillan in the US is a division of St Martin's Press LLC, 175 Fifth Avenue, New York, NY 10010.

Palgrave Macmillan is the global academic imprint of the above companies and has companies and representatives throughout the world.

Palgrave® and Macmillan® are registered trademarks in the United States, the United Kingdom, Europe and other countries.

ISBN 978–0–230–34696–3

This book is printed on paper suitable for recycling and made from fully managed and sustained forest sources. Logging, pulping and manufacturing processes are expected to conform to the environmental regulations of the country of origin.

A catalogue record for this book is available from the British Library.

A catalog record for this book is available from the Library of Congress.

10   9   8   7   6   5   4   3   2   1
22   21   20   19   18   17   16   15   14   13

Contents

Diagrams and Tables

Diagrams

Tables

Foreword

For some time now, I have been becoming increasingly concerned by the amount of time that nurses spend trying to tie down precisely what spirituality is. Has it to do with God? Does it relate to issues of meaning, purpose and love? Is it in fact a concept birthed in nursing fiction? Or is it in fact a vital and often forgotten dimension of nursing practice? All of these positions can be found within the literature and perhaps such conversations are important. But in the end, none of them can claim to have answered the question of what spirituality is or whether it exists or otherwise. Some would say that that is a very good reason for getting rid of spirituality from health-care discourse. If we don't know what it is that we are talking about, then how on earth can we make a claim that it is something that is worthy of attention in terms of policy and practice? There is truth in such a thought if one believes that truth is only to be found in propositions, definitions and things that you can see. But, as we listen to the voices of patients, as we reflect on the experiences of carers as they encounter the pain and suffering of others, issues of meaning, value, purpose, hope and God permeate the conversation like air permeates the alveoli of our lungs. It sometimes feels like such things are the very breath of care and the proper shape of human striving for peace and healing in the midst of suffering and distress. We seem to need spirituality in order to suffer hopefully. Does it matter what we call such deep experiences? Perhaps it does. The language of spirituality may well remain necessary to remind us of those aspects of our caring practices that easily get left behind and overlooked due to shortage of time and our often necessary focus on managing tasks. But perhaps we need to begin to define it from a different perspective; according to what it *does* and what it *means* for patients and nurses rather than what it conceptually may or may not be. When viewed 'from below', spirituality is not a highly complicated concept that is clarified and improved by incessant academic reflection. When viewed from the experience of human suffering, spirituality is discovered when we learn what it means to be with one another in illness and in health. Spirituality is easily encountered as we listen closely to the meanings that patients give to their experiences. It flows smoothly between us as we encounter one another in deep ways; as we catch, if only for a moment, the knowing eye of a person with dementia as they lock into that moment. It races towards us as we hear the person with terminal cancer ask us what their life has meant. It eases its way into conversations within which illness forces carer and cared for to ask why? What does this all mean? What does my family mean to me? Where is my God? Spirituality is found not in the academy, but in the deep processes of everyday caring. Perhaps we need to stop arguing about what spirituality is or whether or not it exists and recognise that the deep experiences that the term 'spirituality' has come to represent are immovable aspects of forms of care that take seriously the wholeness and uniqueness of the other.

Janice Clarke's book begins to move us in this direction. Behind all of the confusion over the nature of spirituality, she tells us to slow down and look at what we do. It is in the everyday practices of love and care – the very fabric of nursing – that spirituality comes to the fore. It is not something that has to be named; it is something that we experience, share and move within. As we engage in the everyday practices of nursing so we encounter the spiritual, not in conceptual form but deeply embedded and embodied in the movements of care that we have come to describe as nursing.

The book is deeply practical, intended to help nurses to see the power of their spiritual practices and to begin to recognise that spirituality is not an esoteric thing that is carried out only by 'religious people', but that it is the very fabric of good nursing care. Janice's spirituality is not immaterial; rather it is embodied, physical and filled with hopeful care. Human beings are embodied souls; creatures who reside in bodies not as separate bodies and souls, but as whole creatures whose physical presence invades the transcendent in ways that are tangible and 'fleshy'. The transcendent remains transcendent, but the transcendent is to be found in the midst of the temporal. Nursing is a spiritual practice which requires to be embodied. This book helps us to envision what that might look like.

John Swinton, RMN, RNMD
Professor of Divinity and Religious Studies,
University of Aberdeen UK.
Honorary Professor of Nursing in the Centre for Advanced
Studies in Nursing and Director of the Centre of Spirituality,
Health and Disability, University of Aberdeen.

Acknowledgements

This book would not have seen the light of day if it had not been for the support of Tim, my husband and my colleagues. Tim for his long-suffering care while I wrote and worried, and my colleagues for putting up with my absence so that I could devote myself to the task. Thank you all.

Introduction

For at least the last 30 years the nursing press has talked about nursing and spirituality as though they go hand in hand. Spiritual care has been a part of nurse training for almost as long, and it is the topic of numerous books, policy papers, articles and websites. It can be found in any policy, guideline or framework about patient care, and spirituality is said to epitomise holistic nursing care and to be at the heart of nursing. Yet, contrary to all of this, successive surveys suggest that nurses say that they don't understand spiritual care, they don't understand how they should do it and they don't feel confident in giving it. The usual answer to this from people who write about spiritual care is that nurses and midwives need more education about spirituality. But the likelihood that more nurses will get onto courses and study days about a topic like spirituality, which many still see as esoteric, when there are so many much more pressing problems with nursing is remote. Against this tide, this book will argue that we have been too complacent in assuming that our model of spiritual care only needs more education to take off in practice. We as scholars of the subject need to take an honest look at the guidance we are giving to nurses, and ask whether we can produce something that is easier to understand and practise and that chimes more with what nurses and the rest of society understand as the core values and practices of nursing and midwifery. In this way, we won't need to introduce extra education to explain it. The problem to be solved is about how something as seemingly esoteric as spirituality, which is believed by most people to have something innately human about it, can be made relevant to a human-focused profession like nursing so that it is a natural part of everyday practice. This book presents just such a solution – a new way to see spiritual care, which has the potential to transform nursing.

A topic like spirituality – which is said to be at the heart of nursing, to epitomise nursing even – cannot be spoken of in isolation from the other key issues which face nursing today. In fact, if spirituality is indeed at the heart of holistic nursing care, as is claimed, it should be able to offer some solution to the crisis which besets nursing today. Complaints about poor nursing care seem to pour daily in a depressingly persistent stream from our newspapers, websites and TVs. They carry a weekly litany of shocking stories of malnutrition, patients left in dirt and squalor, patients feeling humiliated and abused, and outraged relatives. Complaints come from patients organisations, government departments, newspapers, TV programmes and quality improvement agencies (Age UK 2010, Care Quality Commission 2011, Patterson 2011a and The Patients Association 2011).

These stories of neglect, unkindness and inhumanity make most nurses feel ashamed of their profession and any nurse with a conscience should be asking: Where did we go wrong? This book is built on the premise that the answer to spirituality's problem lies in its potential to help the profession solve our other problem which is about poor nursing care.

My interest in this subject and my longing to develop this new way of looking at spiritual care came from the perplexing discovery a few years ago that the articles and books I was reading about 'care' didn't talk about spiritual care and the literature about spiritual 'care' didn't talk about care. I had apparently stumbled on the odd fact that these two big subject areas, which had each been the focus of so much analysis and which each claimed to be at the heart of nursing, had been barely connected. I had assumed that 'spiritual care' was about 'care that was spiritual' when clearly spiritual care was about something else. What this book proposes and explains is a way to bring care and spiritual care together – a mix which has the potential to make caring more relevant and rewarding and to ground the concept of spirituality in everyday acts of nursing and midwifery 'care', truly embedding it in practice. This book takes as a basic premise the idea that if a person is seen as a whole, body and soul combined, then there is a potential for the spiritual dimension to be affected and 'cared for' in the way a person is cared for.

Critics will say this 'new' approach 'is just person-centred care then,' as though that were something derogatory. In reality, spiritual care has never been anything but person-centred care, just as anything that any health care practitioner does should be 'person centred'. One of the ironies about the decline in standards of 'personal' nursing care is that for years nursing has focused itself on the person, and 'person-centred care' has been the principle at the core of every educational initiative and National Health Service (NHS) policy. Evidently it hasn't worked. This book will argue that this is because health care practices, while talking about person-centred care, have actually been diverted away from the person and into a focus on the procedure – away from holism and the true meaning of caring for the whole person, into comprehensiveness, which is a belief that 'everything covered' was the same as holism.

The person-centred care talked about in this book is about caring for the whole 'spiritual person', care which constantly acknowledges that what makes a human a human is that there is a deep part of them – which is somehow related to how peaceful, strong and whole they feel, no matter what they call it – which they wish to have acknowledged and valued. It could be called the spirit. The upsurge in interest in this part of a person, or in spirituality, suggests that society is full of people who are hungry for an acknowledgement of what makes them valuable, what makes them more than a biological machine. At the same time, lives are more fragmented, stressful and demanding, with the numbers of lonely, depressed and marginalised people apparently rising. The complaints about nursing are not just indicative of problems in nursing but might also suggest that everyone in society is more aware of the care that they want and where it is missing. How it feels to be cared for is coming to the foreground of public thinking. Nursing needs to respond to all these demands in society not by adding spirituality to its lists of things to do but by absorbing spirituality into everything that it does so that all care is spiritual. Nursing is perfectly situated to do this work in society. However, it seems that the notions of person-centred care which nursing has depended on up to now have not worked. The approach here is a progression from person-centred care; person-centred care for the new millennium. This is spirit-centred care, care of the whole person which constantly acknowledges their spirituality.

One of the strategies in trying to solve the problems of poor care has been the campaign to reinstate dignity in nursing care (McSherry 2010). To Gadow, a nurse philosopher, the moral aim of caring itself is 'the protection and enhancement of human dignity' (1985, p. 32). So the very idea of dignity is embedded in good care, and spiritual care is about restoring dignity. Thus this approach goes to the heart of the dignity campaign.

This new approach to spiritual care is not an abandonment of the current model of 'spiritual care', but it enhances and rejuvenates it while building on the distinctive and unique care that nurses and midwives give and valuing the ordinary daily tasks of care.

The spiritual care talked about in these pages is tuned into the way nurses and midwives work; it builds on the strengths and opportunities of their role. Nevertheless, there is a great deal in this kind of spiritual care which every other health care professional can also tune into and use. This spiritual care rejects the notion of seeing spirituality as separated from all the other things a nurse or midwife does, as something which has to be added on to an already overcrowded day. It is an approach based on the two biggest parts of the work of nurses and midwives: relationships and physical care.

The only special skills required for this spiritual care are the special skills that any nurse or midwife should have – the special skills that many nurses and midwives are already using daily. This is spiritual care for the fainthearted. Spiritual care has to be like this because every nurse and midwife is required to do spiritual care and so there has to be a way to do it that is within the scope of every nurse and midwife . This is it.

Spirituality should be a subject that inspires nurses and midwives, but sometimes the current approach leaves nurses feeling indifferent and confused. But they become excited when asked about the spirituality in the ordinary tasks they perform all day long, like helping a patient to wash or being with a woman when she's giving birth. In those moments, spirituality changes from being something strange, ambiguous and esoteric to something that is alive and sparkling with possibilities. The idea of nursing itself is reborn from being a series of tasks into being a unique opportunity to really make a difference in a person's life just by being with patients in a caring and meaningful way. At the end of one teaching session I gave which included this approach, a student summed up all I had been hearing over the years when she said, 'this is what I came into nursing for'.

Terms used in the book

The following is some basic information about how this book is written.

Patients

To make for rather smoother writing and reading, the term 'patients' has been used to also mean clients and service users. Sometimes these terms are used separately when it seems more appropriate in the context of the writing.

Nurses

The terms 'nurse' and 'nursing' have been used to mean care assistants as well as mental health and paediatric nurses, and it should be seen as including midwives. On occasion, these terms are expressed separately when the context seems to dictate it. The term 'practitioners' is sometimes used to mean all the above and other health professionals. However, as stated earlier, any health professional will find a lot to interest them and to add to their practice throughout this book.

Gender

The feminine gender words are usually used to reflect the fact that most nurses and midwives are female; however, it should be taken to mean male as well as female practitioners.

Illness

'Illness' has been used as a general term to refer to general and mental illness and results of accidents – in fact, any of the maladies or disturbances which bring a person into contact with the health services. It could also refer to complications of disabilities or conditions which have produced disabilities.

Sources

The ideas referred to in this book come from a range of sources across many disciplines including theology, religious texts, religious studies, sociology, philosophy, psychology and education. This is a deliberate strategy to reflect the fact that nursing has not invented the term 'spirituality' and that the subject should be seen within the context of a long history and centuries of study which nursing has at its disposal to draw on. The approach in this book is based on a wide range of evidence and years of study and reflection. It grew out of doctoral research. As described below, the experiences of patients and practitioners have been drawn upon extensively.

Quotations

There are many quotations in this book. This is deliberate. Because spirituality is, to a large extent, subjective and experiential, it is often understood best by hearing about others' ideas and experiences of it, and the exact words they use are important.

Care and spiritual care are not exact sciences; they are difficult to pin down and explain. So it is often only through the words of people being cared for that we can get to the essence of what spiritual care means to the most important people in our professional lives – patients. For this reason, in parts of this book there are the words of a multitude of people who have given their time to help researchers in studies around the world. I have quoted many of their words in full and I am extremely grateful to them all for sharing their experiences and to the researchers who have undertaken these studies and reflected so deeply on their meaning. These studies – and I have only referred to a few compared to the many available – contain a treasury of riches which tell nurses all they need to know about how to care spiritually. In a three-year degree from which nurses and midwives are launched into very busy jobs, I know that there is little time to explore these jewels, and so I hope that these pages will, as well as being enlightening, also inspire you to go on reading. Much of this research has come from phenomenology, which is (usually) a form of interviewing that gives people the chance to talk about the real essence of the lived experience of being cared for. Nurses and midwives should be very grateful to those scholars who have enriched our profession by using this research method to bring us these gems.

Examples

Throughout the book, there are examples which explain how a particular idea in the text might work in practice. They are either something I have experienced or seen or are fictional but are based on my own experience and knowledge.

'Time to think'

Dotted throughout the book are boxes that suggest that it's time to stop reading and think. These are invitations to reflect on what you've just read and to connect it to your own experience.

A note about myself

My background is in Christianity and so the beliefs and sources I know most about are from Christianity. Every person has a point on which they stand, a history and a culture, and nobody can claim to be completely neutral. Any writer is influenced by their beliefs. However, I have tried as far as I could to include other viewpoints. I have also tried to only present ideas which, although sourced from a particular tradition, I know to resonate across many other traditions and cultures. My aim is to present possibilities which might be found useful to as wide a variety of people as possible, and so I have tried to exclude any concept which I know, from my research, to be severely antithetic to another tradition or culture. Every idea has to come from somewhere.

The book's structure

The book is divided into four parts. Part I explains what spirituality is thought to be. Part II is about a few of the things that influence a person's spirituality. Part III is about spiritual care in relationships and care. Part IV is about spiritual care as part of the personal and physical care that nurses and midwives give.

In Part I, Chapter 1 explores the reasons for the current interest in spirituality and the way it has been talked of in nursing and examines some of the issues and problems with the current approach to spiritual care in the profession. Chapter 2 explains in more detail what a person is thought to be and how their spiritual dimension fits in. There is a discussion of what holism really is and what it is not. Next, the part that the body plays in spirituality will be analysed. The chapter goes on to consider how people relate to each other and explains why ideas like compassion are important, why relationships have anything to do with spirituality and how care could be spiritual. It is in this chapter that the theory of this new approach is elaborated.

In Part II there are four chapters and each explores something that has a big influence on a person's spirituality. There are many subjects that could have been included but there's only space for four, so I've chosen a mixed bag of topics; these are age, illness, mental illness and religion. The first chapter in Part II (Chapter 3) is an exploration of how spirituality is different for the young and the old and some suggestions as to how this might affect their spiritual care. Chapter 4 is a careful look at what it actually means to be ill and to have your life disturbed by pain or disability. Although nurses work with sick people all the time, we don't often think that deeply about how it actually feels to be ill, but in this chapter people speak for themselves about the experience. I am indebted in particular to Michael Stein for these insights, from his study of what it means to be ill. This is followed by Chapter 5, which looks at the role that religion can play in a person's life and why religion is important to a person's spirituality, together with some ideas as to how to include a person's religion in their spiritual care. Chapter 6 in this part connects spirituality to mental illness and examines what mental health professionals say about how religion and spirituality influence their patients, especially in relation to depression and psychosis.

The first chapter of Part III (Chapter 7) will take you to the subject of relationships in nursing and midwifery, with a look at what care is and what patients say about being cared for. The reader is taken into the area of relationships, care and comfort and how all nurses can give spiritual care in how they relate, care for and comfort patients. The second chapter of Part III (chapter 8) explores how nurses and midwives can practise spiritual care through presence and empathy. This chapter explores how nurses and midwives can practise spiritual care through presence and empathy. The next chapter (Chapter 9) goes into the difficult topic of talking about spirituality with a discussion of the place of spiritual assessment and a few hints about how you can introduce the topic of spirituality to patients who might want to talk.

The first chapter of Part IV (Chapter 10) moves us towards the physical body and how patients say the body feels when it is ill, and a look at how this affects our spiritual well-being. Then the important subject of touch will be delved into in detail in a chapter all of its own (Chapter 11). This is followed by three chapters (Chapters 12, 13 and 14) examining the spiritual care involved in helping someone to move, bathing someone and helping with mealtimes and eating. These last three chapters bring the rest of the book together to apply what you've learnt to practical situations. These may not be situations every nurse will use every day, but I hope it will give you ideas about how the same principles can be applied to your own practice.

Regretfully there are many areas of spiritual care that time and space have not allowed me to include here, areas in which the spiritual care possibilities are enormous and very important, such as learning disability and dementia. I am confident that nurses working in these areas will see for themselves how these principles can be applied to their work.

I hope you will see as you work your way through this book that what you are reading is a unique way of thinking about spiritual care, although it is a way based on very ancient ideas and principles and on knowledge that all of us already have within us.

Part I
Introducing Spirituality

1 What is spirituality?

Introduction

Interest in spirituality has swept through society touching almost everything in its path. There is hardly an aspect of modern life which it hasn't been associated with. It seems like almost everywhere you look these days, in politics, economics, management, education, health care, art, music, science or business, there is a mention of spirituality. In particular, from a very early stage in this new awakening, it has been linked to health and it was quickly adopted by nursing as an aspect of patient care that ought to be addressed. This chapter will explore what this spirituality is about and how it is linked to nursing and answer the question of how nurses and midwives should best address the spirituality issue in practice.

Spirituality in history and religion

The term 'spirituality' comes from the Latin *spiritualitas* and spiritual is from *spiritualis*. These terms themselves are derived from the Greek *pneuma* meaning spirit and *pneumatikos* meaning spiritual. *Pneuma* also means wind or breath in Greek (Sheldrake 2007).

At first the word was used exclusively in Christianity and gradually came to be used by other religions, but it is not a word that has been used outside theological circles until recently. The word 'spirituality' has been rediscovered by modern society to express something that many people feel has been lost, but the idea of spirituality has always been present in religions because spiritual beliefs are the bedrock of religious belief.

Modern spirituality

Reasons for the current interest

One of the reasons for the explosion of interest in spirituality is called 'the subjective turn' (Heelas and Woodhead 2005). Past generations have tended to live their lives according to norms imposed from outside themselves rather than by relying on their own experiences and feelings to provide a compass for their life. But there has been a turn towards realising that you could be master of your own life and decide your own values. We take this for granted now, but it is a relatively new phenomenon. Heelas and Woodhead (2005) call this the development of an inner subjective life and they see it as being as sacred in its own way as the religious life which used to hold sway in society. This 'something' which needs to be sought and held onto could be perceived as a wholly internal source of strength (which might be called a spirit) or be seen as connected to something outside which might be powerful and immaterial but would not necessarily be called God and would not necessarily be connected to any religion. However it is perceived, the 'inner' person has to some extent replaced religion and perhaps replaced God to many people, and it has caused people to cease looking outside themselves for guidance or inspiration. This increased awareness of an inner self has happened alongside a shift from an emphasis on the community to an emphasis on the uniqueness and importance of the individual, so that spirituality has come to be seen as something which is mostly internal and introverted. Although it may depend on relationships it is experienced by most people as something internal, it is now part of our general understanding of life that individuals 'deserve' to be happy and fulfilled and to have their inner selves fed and nurtured; we have become defined by our inner needs (Walter 1985). Today people expect that their education, government and health services will not only provide systems that give a satisfactory and safe service but that they will also provide personal fulfilment and give individuals the opportunity to reach their full potential. It may be that it is this growth in emphasis on individual personal fulfilment and nurturing the needy inner self that has sparked off the interest in spirituality.

A revitalised idea of the person

In conjunction with the movements in society towards awareness of the inner self and the fulfilment of individuals, there is also a realisation that the kind of society we have is not nurturing people as it should. There is a perception that society is ordered as though human beings were units without souls, and there is a nagging worry that this somehow doesn't take account of the whole person. There was a moment when people thought that they no longer needed ideas about the sacred in their lives, religion appeared to be vanishing and it seemed that peace and contentment could come without the need for the spiritual. In recent decades however it has become clear that religion is not disappearing and some religions in some parts of the world are growing. Some religions are also growing in influence even in modern societies where it was thought that secularisation was going to dominate. People are finding that they are thinking about their soul and they want to include a spiritual dimension in their lives and to have the notion of spirit and soul brought back into concepts about a person in general and they want health-care systems, government, businesses and education to take account of that revitalised idea of the person.

Searching for certainty and strength

When the world looks unstable and threatening or their own lives are uncertain, perhaps because of illness or other major life changes, people find that they need certainty and some source of strength either inside or outside themselves. Although society is now much more affluent with higher standards of living, at least in the West, than previous generations could have dreamt of, there is also the constant worry that the planet is dying and species are disappearing. Increased media and communication means that people are more aware of the greater affluence that others have. Life feels more pressured and faster. People live longer but worry that they may live with more pain and suffering. All these aspects of modern life seem to make it more important to people that they can find a source of strength inside which helps them to find a meaning in life that transcends inequalities, earthquakes, illness and instability, a place within themselves which is stable and sure – a source of strength which will help them to cope with change, uncertainty and injustice. However, today people have to work out again where to find that source of strength. A new language has to be created when people don't want to use the traditional frameworks and narratives to be found in the religions. In this search for a new way of incorporating the spirit back into humanity, the sacred is being sought everywhere. The idea that 'God is within' or that the way to God is through the true self which resides within each person is not a new idea and it has always existed within most religions; the difference is that today many people decide that they don't need religion to access the sacred or to live out ideas about the sacred in their daily life (Tacey 2003).

Spirituality and health care

When people expect their spirit to be taken account of in health care and nurses expect to be holistic and take account of the whole person, it is unsurprising that nursing and health care have adopted the premise of spirituality and decided to incorporate it into its services. Numerous health-care directives and guidelines call for nurses and midwives to address the spiritual dimension (National Institute for Health and Clinical Excellence 2004, NHS Education for Scotland 2009, Nursing and Midwifery Council 2009 and 2010, and others).

A guiding precept for the development of an approach to using spirituality in health care is that it has to be acceptable to people with a wide variety of beliefs and attitudes towards spirituality including complete rejection of the concept altogether. The Royal College of Psychiatrists (2011, p. 7) describes the range of reactions as 'identification with a particular social or historical tradition (or traditions), adoption of a personally defined or personal but undefined spirituality, disinterest, antagonism', which gives some idea of the range of responses required by practitioners. It would be impossible to develop an approach where each element that inspired the model of spirituality is believed in by every patient, but it is important that the resulting guidance should be broadly acceptable. A second precept, as has been mentioned before, is that it should be focused on what spirituality *does* rather than what it *is* because a concept for nursing has to have usefulness to have value. Nursing is a practice profession aimed towards achieving particular aims on behalf of patients and spiritual well-being, for instance, is an aim that can be worked towards.

The debate about definition

There are some human concepts, particularly when they are relatively new, that cannot be defined with the neatness of a scientific theory. This is particularly irksome in systems like health care which is expensive and so has to prove the value of any new idea before it is adopted. Hence, there is a drive to have a definition on which everyone agrees. It has to be said, however, that spiritual care (especially as it is presented in this book) is not an expensive idea to put into practice. It is not dependent on any technology, drug or new building. The idea of spirituality is socially constructed and seems to have an appeal to the general public; it usefully represents notions and longings that are not otherwise represented (Swinton and Pattison 2010), and as such it behoves a service such as nursing to consider whether and how it should be addressed in nursing care. However, the profession should not attempt to expropriate it and pin it down so that lay people can no longer understand it and need to have it explained to them; it is a term in public ownership and scholars have to live with its chaos and ambiguity (Clarke 2009).

Spirituality is inherently a subversive concept which means that it often leads people to kick against the established ways of doing things. It seems to work against some trends in society such as technology, systematisation and materialistic acquisition, and similarly it resists attempts at tight definition. Tight definition can fix in place a single idea of a concept which then sets a particular course in discussions excluding any further debate. Having a concise definition of a tricky concept like spirituality has a seductive attraction because it seems to increase understanding, but this may be an illusion. Such a definition, once it gains momentum, will be pounced on by researchers and writers and quoted so frequently that it will come to seem like the truth instead of only one aspect of the truth. In addition a firm definition would have to be universally applicable to everyone, all beliefs, cultures, religions and professions. Yet researchers looking for such a definition will inevitably view concepts within the framework of their own profession and the people they are researching seldom represent all beliefs. Therefore definitions have tended to be swayed towards particular world views and to represent particular agendas or they become so big and cumbersome in the effort to include all human life that they become impossible to make use of in practice (Clarke 2009). It might be better to think about descriptions of spirituality as marking out an area of thinking about which there is actually little that can easily be concretely described (Swinton and Pattison 2010) but what can be said is that it describes qualities or attitudes which are perceived as missing from modern health-care practice (Swinton and Pattison 2010). Despite the absence of a neat, tight and short definition, there are characteristics or family resemblances which recur with regularity and which have remained remarkably stable over decades in the literature on spirituality in health and nursing. There seems to be virtually no difference between perceptions of spirituality now compared to a few decades ago.

The most important question about spirituality in relation to health care is to ask, does it have a use that can be turned to value in health care so that patients benefit from practitioners paying any attention to it. So it may be that a vague definition is fine, but it must be useful (Swinton and Pattison 2010). This book therefore will not base itself on any one definition but rather, in the 'spirit' of public service, will utilise all the various themes and understandings of spirituality in the public and professional gaze.

Spirit

Spirituality is derived from the idea of spirit which many believe dwells in everyone. Swinton (2001, p. 14) calls it 'the essential life force that undergirds, motivates and vitalizes human existence', spirituality being how over time people and their communities have responded to the idea or experience of having a spirit.

Spiritual well-being

People seem to perceive that their spirit is capable of change and will affect their feeling about themselves, the state of their emotions and whether they feel well in themselves or not. This is how Ellison, who has researched how spiritual 'well-being' can be measured, describes it:

> It is the *spirit* of human beings which enables and motivates us to search for meaning and purpose in life, to seek the supernatural or some meaning which transcends us, to wonder about our origins and our identities, to require mortality and equity. It is the spirit which synthesizes the total personality and provides some sense of energizing direction and order. The spiritual dimension does not exist in isolation from the psyche and the soma, but provides an integrative force. It affects and is affected by our physical state, feelings, thoughts and relationships. If we are spiritually healthy we will feel generally alive, purposeful and fulfilled, but only to the extent that we are psychologically healthy as well. The relationship is bi-directional because of the intricate intertwining of these two parts of the person.
>
> (Ellison 1983, pp. 331–2)

Ellison suggests here that the spirit is what integrates and synthesises, providing order and direction. He endorses the idea that the spirit is connected to the mind (psyche) and the body (soma) and it interacts with our thoughts, emotions, emotions, physical state and relationships.

Spiritual well-being is often talked about in terms of having resources which enable coping in adversity. Inner strength is a feature and is related to inner strength which is also characterised as a personal resource which contributes to well-being and helps people to overcome challenges and adversity and accept change as inevitable (Lundman et al. 2011). People with inner strength feel connected to family, friends, society and nature; they usually believe that there is a spiritual dimension to life and are able to transcend their own self. Having inner strength also seems to ensue from being able to find meaning in life despite setbacks and adversity (Lundman et al. 2011).

Spirituality

Spirituality refers to all the ways in which the spirit expresses itself outwardly in the ideas and philosophies and beliefs and personality of the person into the world. It refers to the values, beliefs and attitudes that exist in the world, because of the presence of the spirit in people. So while the spirit is unknowable, spirituality is more visible and it can be directly experienced and spoken about. John Swinton describes here the dichotomy between the mystery of 'spirit' and the groundedness of spirituality:

> While the human *spirit* may be deeply mysterious, pointing as it does towards aspects of reality that are deep, unfathomable and transcendent, *spirituality* is a human activity that attempts to express these profound experiences and inner longings in terms that are meaningful for the individual.
>
> (Swinton 2001, p. 21)

Spirituality is contextual; it is influenced by beliefs, culture, personal history, economics and profession, to mention just a few factors which affect it. Consequently there will be some ways in which a person's beliefs about spirituality will be like other people's, because they share a culture or a religion and some ways in which they will be unique, because each person has a particular history and combination of experiences that have influenced them.

The themes in spirituality

Spirituality and spiritual well-being are fluid ideas which people struggle to describe and which feel personal to them. Nevertheless when people are asked about what they think spirituality is, there are repeated and constant themes of 'transcendence, unfolding mystery, connectedness, meaning and purpose in life, higher power and relationships' (Tanyi 2002, p. 502).

Connection

Connection, relationship, communication and harmony are all themes which patients and nurses relate to spirituality. Connection may be to parts of oneself, connection between people, connection between a person and nature, or connection to the universe, God or any higher power. People seem to see the quality of their connections or relationships as being reflected in and reflecting their spiritual well-being. The spiritual dimension is called a connecting, dynamic and unifying force which works within a person to give a feeling of peace and harmony and helps them to relate better to other people or to a God or other spiritual entity or force. Integrating and connecting are similar concepts and one is often talked about as leading to the other so that Goddard suggests the term 'integrative energy' to describe spirituality as something which 'pervades, unites and directs all human dimensions'(1995, p. 810). Similarly a study by Hungelmann et al. (1996), which involved 31 interviews and 150 hours of observation with the aim of determining the defining characteristics of spiritual well-being, also linked it to connection and relationship coming to this description which include dynamism and growth in the idea of connection.

> Spiritual well-being is a sense of harmonious interconnectedness between self, others/nature, and Ultimate Other, which exists throughout and beyond time and space. It is achieved through a dynamic and integrative growth process which leads to a realisation of the ultimate purpose and meaning of life.
>
> (Hungelmann et al. 1996, p. 263)

Van Ness (1996, p. 5) talks about spirituality as a quest for relationships that are optimal with what is authentic, calling spirituality 'the quest for attaining an optimal relationship between what one truly is and everything that is'. A concept analysis on spirituality found that all the terms associated with spirituality seemed to be linked to relationships of some description (Goldberg 1998). The theologian Stephen Pattison says that the need for relationships and attachments seems to be indisputably essential for human beings to thrive such that it should be central to how we understand what people see as important to them and therefore should be central to any understanding of spirituality (Pattison 2010), while McSherry and Jamieson (2011) in their large online survey of UK nurses found that over 70 per cent of more than 4,000 nurses thought that the need for love and harmony was an important spiritual need.

All of this suggests that people seem to feel the need for connection with other human beings around them at a deeper level than personality and common interest. The idea of each person having a spirit or a spiritual dimension which connects with others has often been called upon to explain how people may be able to find deep connections with each other and why they seem to want to connect, relate and integrate, in order to get to a state of spiritual well-being.

Transcendence

Spirituality is also called the dimension that enables someone to be aware of and feel connected to something more powerful than themselves, a higher power, a God or a powerful spiritual energy which fills the world. A person may believe that a power outside them can help them to cope, which is how many people feel about God. If they feel they can connect with something outside themselves, just doing that may give them inner 'spiritual' strength that can help them to find the perspective they need to cope with whatever they are facing. However, a power outside yourself can also be experienced as part of yourself. People may talk of spiritual experiences as being transcendent.

Another way the term 'transcendence' can be used is when a person wants to understand the situation they find themselves in the middle of, they need to know it's boundaries and get an idea of its extent. This is only possible by seeing it as a whole and getting a perspective on it from outside, getting above and outside it and so 'transcending' the situation. Transcending the situation they are in can also mean to 'rise above it', in the sense that they overcome it by not letting it beat them down. This could be a way of coping with illness so that it doesn't take over their life; the ability to do this is often related to having a kind of spiritual strength. Transcending the situation can make a problem seem more surmountable and it may be the presence of 'spirit' which as Speck says here, enables us to perform this transcending act.

> spirituality may be described as a vital essence of our lives that often enables us to transcend our circumstances and find new meaning and purpose, and that can foster hope.
>
> (Speck 2005, p. 28)

Spirituality, with or without God

Whether a person believes in a supernatural power outside themselves or not may be central to how they understand their own
spirituality. For people who believe in God, a relationship with
God may be definitive of having a spirit and spiritual well-being.
However, many people do not believe in God but they do believe
in some non-material force or transcendent force which exists in
nature.

A person's beliefs and their world view may influence how they
find meaning in difficult times as well as defining their values and
influencing the decisions they make. Someone who doesn't believe
in any religion can still believe in some kind of transcendent, non-
material power, energy or influence in their life, which they may
or may not call God. These people might describe themselves as
spiritual but not religious. They do recognise some transcendent
'other' but are not interested in pursuing a religion. Piles (1990)
argued that it is only the fact of a relationship with a transcendent 'other' which differentiates spiritual needs from psychosocial
needs (Piles 1990). However, 20 years on from this, the concept of spirituality has developed in such a way in the United
Kingdom especially, that very many people define themselves as
'spiritual' who do not believe in any kind of God or transcendent
power at all. One such person is Andre Comte-Sponville (2007)
who believes in something 'absolute' but doesn't believe that it is
God (p. 137). He believes that nature is all there is, and there is
no supernatural. However, he very firmly believes in spirituality.
To Comte-Sponville, spirit is the power to think; it is his being
(p. 135). Similarly, the term 'sacred' is often only associated with
religion and God but it actually means something which is set
apart from ordinary life and venerated, like something absolute,
like a sacred trust. Van Hooft (2002) also describes a form of spirituality which doesn't depend on metaphysics when he says that the
mystery and infinity people seek can be found in our encounters
with others in relationships.

So, within this world view, it is entirely possible to be spiritual
and live a spiritual life or aim to have spiritual well-being, without
belonging to a religion or even believing in God. For instance, an
atheist could say that respect for the things that affect their selfhood is sacred to them, and so to be treated carelessly or abusively

will affect their spiritual well-being. Heelas and Woodhead (2005) see the modern focus on the person and their own subjective self as in itself being sacred therefore also associating spirituality with something considered sacred, while avoiding the idea that it has to do with something religious or even non-material.

The huge range of beliefs that makes up mankind defies categorisation. Not only are they various but they are variable and may change with illness. Beliefs often defy description even by the people who hold them, so that often people will categorise themselves in a way that seems to contradict what they say they believe. For instance, someone may say they are an atheist, when they actually mean they don't belong to any religion. A Christian may announce that they believe in reincarnation. A devout Moslem may find that in illness they need their children more than they need their mullah. Someone who regularly argues against religion may find comfort and peace sitting in a church. Therefore categories of belief have to be seen as highly elastic and treated with caution. Particularly when people are in situations of change and flux, beliefs that once seemed solid can start to look fragile or even absurd. This makes it important that nurses use spirituality in their practice in such a way that they do not fix patients' beliefs in time, in documents and in their mind and can respond flexibly to each moment in each encounter.

Meaning

This theme is probably the most consistent across the range of beliefs existing about spirituality. Martsolf and Mickley (1998) cited 'meaning' as one of the most significant attributes of spirituality found in nursing theories and the same could probably be said today. Meraviglia (1999) in her analysis of spirituality in the literature likewise notes that spirituality as a 'new sense of meaning' is a common description. Govier (2000) sees the nurse's role in spiritual care as helping 'those who are suffering to reflect upon and find meaning in their experiences' Greasley et al. (2001), writing about spirituality in mental health care, using focus groups amongst carers, service users and mental health-care workers, found they believed that 'spiritual care related to the acknowledgement of a person's sense of meaning and purpose to life', and there are many other examples.

If life has meaning, it is more fulfilling, adversity is easier to cope with, and at the end of our life we will have felt it well spent. If people know why they are doing anything, it adds depth to it, gives it a purpose and makes it more enjoyable and easier, so that in times of sickness and trouble, people may look for the meaning in what has happened, and often cannot find it. There may be no answer to why a person has cancer and a reason for carrying on may, for many people, have to be found away from the search for a reason. Aside from reasons, meaning could be found in having depth and purpose in what we do in life, which seems to give life itself more depth than living it on the surface.

Many nurses have referred to Victor Frankl (1905–1997), a psychotherapist who reached his understanding of the importance of meaning in life during his experiences in a concentration camp. He believed that finding a meaning in suffering helped a person to cope with it. Frankl was very specific that what helped you find meaning were the beliefs you held about life and your attitude towards the burden you had to cope with. He said that meaning can be found in different ways: '(1) by creating a work or doing a deed; (2) by experiencing something or encountering someone; and (3) by the attitude we take toward unavoidable suffering'. He expanded on the nature of the work, the deed or the encounter which will give meaning by saying that it was necessary to be human to transcend your own self and look outward to the world. He said:

> Being human always points, and is directed, to something, or someone, other than oneself be it a meaning to fulfil or another human being to encounter.
>
> (1984 p. 133)

and by experiencing (2) Frankl said that he meant experiencing,

> goodness, truth and beauty by experiencing nature and culture or last but not least, by experiencing another human being in his very uniqueness by loving him.
>
> (Frankl 1984, p. 133)

These quotes suggest that finding meaning was not only about believing in something but that what you believed and how you lived mattered; to Frankl it seems anything will not do. He believed that relationships and meetings with other people can give life meaning and he also seems to say that even in the face of the worst suffering, each person has the internal spiritual freedom to choose his attitude towards it. The key is that you don't always have to see yourself as being at the mercy of your circumstances. Even when the circumstances can't be changed, the way you feel about it can. As Frankl says, 'When we are no longer able to change a situation – just think of an incurable disease such as an inoperable cancer – we are challenged to change ourselves' (Frankl 1984, p. 135).

The theologian Paul Tillich (1886–1965) is also well known for saying that it is not only having meaning but what those meanings are, that matter, and that thinking about the serious and ultimate concerns of life, and not just about pleasure will be what gives ultimate meaning (Clarke 2006a). Reflections on the thoughts of these two authors suggest that it is not only having meaning that makes a difference but also what that meaning is. It also suggests that someone can work to create meaning and to change their attitude to suffering and it is encounters with the people around them that might create meaning and be the catalyst for other meanings to be made.

Spirituality is often experienced as consciously putting in the effort to move towards a goal as Schneiders emphasises here: the effort of consciously trying to think less about ourselves but to look outward as Frankl says above. Schneiders definition of spirituality is from a survey of theology literature:

> The experience of consciously striving to integrate one's life in terms not of isolation and self-absorption but of self-transcendence towards the ultimate value one perceives.
>
> (Schneiders 1989, p. 684)

Sims and Cook who are psychiatrists sum up all these things as existing within a person and within communities, seeing relationship as fundamental to the concept.

> a distinctive, potentially creative, and universal dimension of human experience arising both within the inner subjective awareness of individuals and within communities, social groups

and traditions. It may be experienced as a relationship with that which is intimately 'inner' immanent and personal, within the self and others, and/or as relationship with that which is wholly 'other', transcendent and beyond the self. It is experienced as being of fundamental or ultimate importance and is thus concerned with matters of meaning and purpose in life, truth, and values.

(Sims and Cook 2009, p. 4)

The themes of connection, transcendence and meaning are linked together by the thread of relationship. They all contain elements of relating, integration and moving outside the self towards the world and other people.

Embodiment and spirituality

Ellison's description of spiritual well-being explains that the spiritual dimension is not isolated from the body but is influencing and influenced by how we feel, think and relate (Ellison 1983). The spirit and therefore spirituality are inextricably bound to body as well as mind, yet it is regularly talked about only in terms of mental and emotional processes. The idea of spirituality as thoroughly embodied has been embedded in much religious doctrine, but as in the rest of society, the association between the spirit and the body has been historically neglected, and religions are seen as treating the body as something to be controlled and its demands submerged if spiritual progress was to be made. But the reality as spirituality is lived for most religious people is that they are deeply engaged with the body in their worship and everyday practices (McGuire 2007). Across all religions and secular spiritualities, spiritual practices involve the body. In meditation and yoga and in religious worship, kneeling, prostration, making the sin of the cross and bowing your head are all bodily practices that people use to connect themselves with the spiritual. McGuire (2007) cites *pranayama* as the epitome of an embodied spiritual practice where the breath is controlled rhythmically so as to develop spiritual strength. Music is used in most religions like plainchant and singing in the Christian tradition and drumming in Native American religion. Dancing in the form of the whirling dervishes is essential to Sufism and belly dancers see their practice as spiritual.

Similarly art is made physically and experienced and responded to using the senses and it has always been used to promote and maintain spiritual development (Kraus 2009). Icons are essential to Eastern Orthodox Christians for the very reason that they emphasise an essential aspect of Christian theology which is that the body and the whole material world are spiritual.

Spirituality and religion

There has been a tendency to contrast spirituality and religion with religion often compared negatively with spirituality (Zinnbauer et al. 1999, Clarke 2006b). However, the two are very closely related and understanding religion may even help in understanding spirituality and vice versa. For instance, spirituality is defined by Pargament (1997) as the search for the sacred, and connection with the sacred could be said to be central to religions. The longings which lead people to religion are the same longings that lead people to spirituality. Religion is one form of spirituality and each religion has a distinctive set of spiritual beliefs. Religions have developed when spiritual beliefs have coalesced over centuries and become institutionalised. Spiritual beliefs have been represented in religion as ritual symbols, as narratives and for guidance within a particular world view so that they can be embedded and lived out in the experience of daily life. All the themes mentioned above related to spirituality exist in religions. Therefore it is not surprising that people have sought religion in order to live out the spiritual dimension of themselves. For instance, relationship is essential to the person, essential to spirituality and is the central theme of Christianity (Pattison 2010). The oldest religions have been studying for centuries questions like – What is a person? How can you live a happy life? How can you live in tune with nature? How can you live a spiritual life with a physical body? Does compassion matter; and if it does, Why? What kinds of love are there? How do you love someone you don't like? How can illness and disaster be lived with? and many more similar questions. These are the kind of questions that people have grappled with for centuries inside and outside religion, and it means that religions can be one source of knowledge about spirituality. For many people, their religion is fundamental to how they experience the world – so it cannot be ignored by nurses and midwives. Recognition of this fact has increased in recent years (Department of Health 2009). But also, the divide between secular and religious spiritual beliefs is so porous that people can drift into and out of religions as and when they need them and especially in times of change such as illness.

The current approach to spiritual care in nursing

Nursing care is organised around the nursing process, which is a problem-based, rationalistic and mechanistic system and so naturally this has become the way spiritual care is spoken of and introduced to nurses (McSherry 2006). At the root of the nursing process is the notion that patients have needs or problems and the nurse's role is to meet those needs or solve the problems. Consequently spirituality is spoken of most often in terms of spiritual needs, which are identified by assessment, and care is implemented on that basis. McSherry and Ross (2010) have modified their approach recently to be still systematic but no longer use the word 'process'. Needs identifying systems have become ingrained in our culture, encouraged in health care by the ubiquitous authority of Maslow's pyramidal structure which all nurses are probably familiar with (Walter 1985); most issues can be converted into sets of needs to be met or problems to be solved. Assess, identify goals, plan, implement and evaluate has become a mantra which has proved very successful at systematising the complexity of planning care. However, whilst recognising that people have needs, the notion of 'needs' seems to have become definitive of a person's spirituality. This is detrimental to the relational dimension of spirituality not only because it dominates, leaving little room for other approaches, but also because seeing a person as 'needy' is not conducive to positive relationships. People are more than sets of needs.

Another challenge for the current approach is in education. It is well recognised that while most nurses now know about spirituality, they are unsure how to use it in practice or they find doing it too difficult (Noble and Jones 2010, McSherry and Jamieson 2011). McSherry has identified many of the barriers to including the current model of spirituality in practice such as lack of privacy and embarrassment in talking about spiritual needs, and the emotional demands and the fear this invokes (McSherry 2006). The most commonly repeated barrier cited by nurses is lack of confidence to give spiritual care because they feel poorly educated on the subject specifically in how to assess spiritual needs, despite access to numerous journal papers and books about it (McSherry and Jamieson 2011). Realistically, time and privacy are at a premium, education is expensive and staffing levels are so pared down that staff cannot be released for education, so that these barriers are not likely to disappear (Moss et al. 2011).

In addition, spiritual care has come to be seen as an 'add on' to the care which is already given; and with most nurses working under an already intolerable burden of work and responsibilities, spirituality has become a marginalised aspect of care. It may have become more embedded in nursing rhetoric, but it has not become embedded in nursing practice. Nurses very strongly feel that spirituality is something that they should be addressing and it is generally agreed that they should be providing it, but large numbers feel they are only sometimes meeting spiritual needs (McSherry and Jamieson 2011). The time is right, therefore, to examine whether there is a different way of thinking about spiritual care.

Appropriateness of the current approach for spirituality

Nurses tend to cite one barrier as the embarrassment and difficulty in talking about spirituality and especially spiritual assessment. This begs the question whether such a rational, systematic problem-solving approach should be used for such a subjective, irrational, mysterious and personal notion as the spiritual dimension. While education will help, it is unlikely to entirely resolve this issue. One of the dilemmas with assessment tools is that they either tend to be too focused on religion or too focused on psychosocial matters (Clarke 2009), each of which are inappropriate and perplexing for nurses and clients. Religion appears in assessment tools because these questions are preferable to trying to ask questions about 'spirituality' which, detached from its links to religion, is equally mystifying. However, *in action*, it is understood as the added something that makes a person more than the sum of their parts; it makes holism make sense. Studies with patients, some of which are mentioned below, show that they see spirituality as more palpable in what someone does and how they are, than in the answers to questions. These pressures on spiritual care to become a system of assessment, problem solving and measurement could easily damage such a subversive, amorphous and relational concept as spirituality, submerging and reducing it to the point where it is lost. As the sociologist Walter contends, in his argument against this 'routinisation' of spiritual care:

> The great spiritual teachers of the world would surely turn in their graves to hear spirituality turned into a discourse of clients, needs, goals, care plans and outcomes!
>
> (Walter 1997, p. 27)

Appropriateness for patients

Arguably viewing persons through the lens of their 'needs' and 'problems' could be seen as objectifying the person; treating them as an object to be analysed rather than as a subject in their own world to whom you have to relate in order to learn personal things about them. The incorporation of spirituality into the realm of nursing as just another area to be exposed, assessed, planned for and evaluated could be seen as another advance in the process which Nettleton calls 'the creeping medicalization of phenomena' (1995, p. 157) where more and more of the patient and their personal world is laid bare and claimed by medical 'experts' to be turned into pathology – a process evident in the diagnosis of spiritual distress, where the language of disease is applied to normal spiritual processes and changes (North American Nursing Diagnosis Association 2012). A second reason to question the appropriateness of the current approach to spirituality for patients is that patients are mostly concerned with being cared for and the current approach has nothing to say to critics of the quality of ordinary nursing care. Another reason is that, as will be shown here, patients themselves seem to see spiritual care in terms of how caring nurses are, rather than whether they are able to talk about spirituality.

Appropriateness for nursing

The current approach could be said to *divide* people into needs and problems, and *separate* their spiritual dimension from the rest of their being. This is paradoxical, when spirituality *and* nursing are both about connections, relationships and integration. While the current approach depends on nurses *talking* to patients, spirituality is actually *embodied* and nursing and midwifery are intrinsically *physical* activities dealing with embodied beings; yet physicality appears barely to enter into spiritual care as it is portrayed in the literature. While talking is very important, there is much more to nursing than talk. The people that nurses care for may not have the cognitive skills to process ideas about spirituality, let alone to talk about them, nor to talk about spiritual care. They may have dementia or a learning disability, and for them a talk-based spiritual care may not fit.

The fact that the current approach is not focused on the activities that nurses do best which are caring, body-work and relationships means that they are not using their own nursing skills to give spiritual care and seem to be forced to adapt themselves to another way which may be more suited to the predominantly 'talking' role of the chaplain and the counsellor. This is disempowering and anxiety-provoking for nurses. As Noble and Jones discovered when they interviewed a group of nurses where they found 'feelings of guilt, inadequacy and stress at being unable to assess and address patients spiritual needs', and 'a recurring concern... was the fear and anxiety around the perceived lack of skills in spiritual assessment' (Noble and Jones 2010, p. 568). Spiritual care, as it is written about, is dominated by the notion of nurse-initiated discussions, but the nurses in Noble and Jones (2010) study felt that spiritual care should be guided by patients, and Taylor and Mamier's (2005) study with cancer patients showed that what they wanted most was not to talk, but humour and a quiet place to think. These patients didn't particularly want to be listened to while they talked about their spiritual concerns and they definitely didn't want interventions such as nurses encouraging them to talk by suggesting drawing or writing about spirituality. Conco (1995) found that patients described spiritual care as taking time, being present and available, using touch and giving good nursing care. What these patients wanted most was a sense of connection. Conco's conclusion was that they were basically describing the characteristics of care. Tanyi et al.'s study (2006) also found that patients saw spiritual care mostly as displaying genuine caring, with patience, kindness, listening, smiling and giving information amongst other caring skills. While some patients valued being able to talk about specific spiritual concerns, many didn't, and for those for whom it mattered, it wasn't uppermost in their minds as a way to receive spiritual care. In McSherry and Jamieson's (2011) study, while nurses felt that they were unable to provide spiritual care, they also believed that spiritual care was mostly a case of helping people to have hope, being cheerful, listening having respect for privacy and dignity, giving support and reassurance and having relationships, which is ordinary nursing care. This seems to mean that they could not recognise the spiritual care in what they were already doing. Studies such as these suggest that there is a gap between what patients say they want and what nurses have been led to believe they should have. There is also a profound lack of confidence amongst nurses about their ability to give spiritual care and a lack of recognition of the spirituality in the care they are already giving. How much more could they give if they had more confidence in their own nursing skills.

Nurses seem to have been led to emulate the chaplain, the doctor, the social worker and the counsellor, probably because these were the role models closest at hand in this new sphere of spiritual care. But nurses have their own unique opportunities and style with which to meet a patient's need for connection, relationship, love, transcendence and meaning-making, by the care that they themselves give.

Another vision of spiritual care

Alongside the approach to spiritual care discussed above there has always run another thread which is to do with how the nurse is, how she communicates, uses her presence, values people, acts compassionately and is of service to the patient, and a few authors have explored this (McSherry 2006, Puchalski 2010, Baldacchino 2011), some emphasising it more than others (NHS Education for Scotland 2009). Swinton (2001), for instance, describes spiritual care as practical wisdom and sees it as a way of working with patients rather than a separate aspect of care and Bradshaw (1997) has called for a new approach to spiritual care which acknowledges that it is about *how* we care. However, these skills do not predominate, and are usually only seen as facilitating a talking or a nursing process approach by encouraging patients to disclose their needs. While creating relationships where patients feel free to talk about themselves is certainly part of spiritual care, it is also the relationships themselves and the care, love, warmth, presence, touch, competence, assurance and security they can provide which should be recognised *to be* spiritual care, in and of itself. It is this issue that the remainder of this book will be about.

This way of seeing spiritual care resonates with the notion of therapeutic nursing, which McMahon and Pearson (1998, p. 7) call 'the practice of those nursing activities which have a healing effect or those which result in a movement towards health or wellness'. One category of therapeutic nursing is the nurse–patient relationship, led by the idea that nursing relationships could in themselves be healing and so therapeutic and not only as a facilitating, organising or enabling force for other therapeutics. Realising the power of nursing in this way and recognising the spiritual effects that our relationships could have on patients could help to raise the confidence of nurses and midwives in these times of increasing criticism and help them find meaning in what they do; a meaning which seems to have become obscured for many nurses. Healing means much more than cure, and an approach which has the potential to help people feel whole again, even with the presence of disease and disability, could indeed be seen as healing.

Isolation and loneliness are common feelings in illness (Stein 2008). Feeling a connection with nurses can help patients to feel they are still part of the world. But spiritual well-being is also about inner connections and feeling that the parts of yourself are in harmony and not jangling together disconnected and chaotic. Connection creates integration and integration leads to feelings of completeness and wholeness. Connection, integration and wholeness are all qualities which are at risk of disappearing when the isolation, dis-integration, and brokenness of illness, change and pain set in. To feel part of something bigger than themselves may help to give patients the perspective they need to put their illness into perspective and to find a place for the new or changed person to grow. The security of care and connectedness could enable patients to transcend their present situation to explore the possibilities for finding a renewed purpose in their life and in their illness.

Illness, accident and disability change the body, and new relation-ships with the body have to be formed in order to find wholeness again. Care-full touch and attention to dignity and comfort which nurses can use in all the physical tasks of nursing can help patients to find assurance of their innate value and move people to feeling at home in their body again.

New meanings and purpose cannot be given, they can only be found; and nurses, by their presence throughout the day, are able to create relationships and environments within which patients can explore their new situation and find new directions. Finding mean-ing, rather than being the starting point of spirituality, is the end point of a journey and spirituality is often experienced as a journey, a journey with companions. Having connections, feeling valued, feeling related and integrated, being able to transcend the present situation by having a task or some work to do which gives you a goal in life and helps you stay connected to the world, having pos-itive encounters with other people and being able to choose the attitude you are going to take to the situation you are in may all lead to being able to find meaning in the situation you are in or at least a reason to live each day. The beliefs that a person carries with them are part of them. Helping people to connect or recon-nect with those beliefs and live them out is part of valuing a person as well as a way of helping them to access that which can give them strength and support in the task of finding new meanings.

Nurses are different because they are never focused on only one part of the person or one therapy; our remit is to care and we are orientated towards more than just the outcomes of therapy. We are present throughout the day, every day – when the patient is in the bath, on the bedpan and leaning over the vomit bowl – in the most intimate and private acts that keep a body going. We have a privi-leged relationship with patients which allows us to be with patients when they are at their most exposed and vulnerable. We can do more than hold a patient's hand, we can stroke a back or give a soothing bath. All of this makes the case that nurses have a distinct and unique contribution to make to a patient's spiritual care that is different to the contribution that the chaplain, the social worker, the counsellor or the doctor can make.

The nurse's day is full of personal encounters and how they manage each encounter is the bedrock of the nurses' work and the beginning of spiritual care.

Conclusion

What if nurses can meet patients' spiritual needs for compassion by acting compassionately, for connection, by connecting, for transcendence by together with them transcending the moment they are in. What if? What would that spiritual care look like? What would that nursing care look like?

This chapter has offered some reasons for the interest in spirituality in society in general and explored some of its links with health care. A lot of space has been given to exploring some problems with the way spirituality is currently incorporated into nursing and an alternative way has been suggested. The following pages will go on to examine how a more holistic way of thinking of a person and their spirituality will help to explain why a more relational and embodied way of doing spiritual care makes sense for nursing and midwifery.

2 Body and soul: An integrated person model

Introduction

This chapter will discuss a model of the person to help explain how what nurses do every day is potentially spiritual care. A model can't exactly represent reality but it just helps people to understand reality better. It may be that the reason why we have the current approach to spiritual care and the reason why the current way of viewing person-centred care hasn't produced good care, is because of the model of the person that nurses have been working from.

The most common way of depicting a person and their spirituality is a Venn diagram of three or four slightly overlapping circles of body, mind, spirit and sometimes social or environmental aspects (Malinski 2002) (Diagram 2.1). But what is not usually depicted is whether these parts interact. This is important because, first of all nursing is meant to be holistic and address the 'whole person', so nurses need to know what a whole person is. Secondly it's important because, from the previous chapter, it can be seen that spirituality is so much about connecting and relating, and nursing is so much about the body, that the model nurses use should be able to explain how the spirit, mind and body are connected and related. Scholars of human relating and being have sometimes decried the fact that we don't have an adequate way of viewing how the parts of a person are related to each other in a holistic way. For instance McGuire, a sociologist of religion, says:

> We must reconceptualise mind, body and society, not as merely connected, but as deeply interpenetrating, meshed as a near unitary phenomenon.
>
> (McGuire 1990, p. 285)

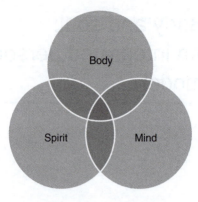

Diagram 2.1   The usual way of depicting how body, mind and spirit relate: A basic Venn diagram

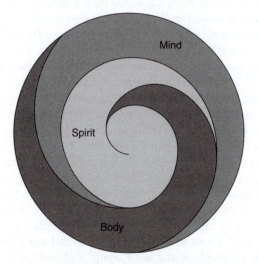

Diagram 2.2   Spiral integrated model of body, mind and spirit showing overlaying dynamic and interpenetrating parts with constant movement between each part

The model presented here will try to take up McGuire's challenge by showing that a person is made up of deeply penetrating parts which together form a unity. This is depicted here as a spiral (Diagram 2.2) with body, mind and spirit enmeshed and immersed in each other, embracing each other in a dynamic whirl. A person is a complicated entity and can't be summed up very easily, but a working model can be created which is useful for practice. Most nursing theories and models were created before the time when there was much discussion about spirituality – and so they either don't include spirituality or theorists have revised their earlier ideas and added it on (Malinski 2002). With the rise in interest in spirituality, nursing theories have had to adapt themselves to the new spirituality and the idea of what a person is that nurses currently work with do not necessarily fit with contemporary ideas of a person.

The model nurses use should resonate with the instincts and knowledge that nurses and midwives have about a person and be acceptable to the generality of faiths and beliefs and cultures in the patients nurses come across. While there are many different conceptualisations of the person and the body embedded in faiths and cultures across the world, models such as this one described here, with the elements of integration, holism and microcosm, are common, while the opposite idea, dualism, which sees more separation between body and mind seems to be more embedded in thinking in the modern West (Scheper-Hughes and Lock 1987). Many of the ways that we have of talking about what a person is and the relationship of spirituality to what it means to be a person come from religions and theology. This is understandable when you consider that this is the main subject matter of religions and theology. To choose to ignore these ways because they grew out of a particular religion is unwise because it cuts us off from a huge part of human history and wisdom. This is also the view of Kaufmann (Translator of Buber and writer of the prologue to *I and Thou*) who said:

> why use religious terms? Indeed, it might be better not to use them because they are always misunderstood. But what other terms are there? We need a new language, and new poets to create it, and new ears to listen to it. Meanwhile if we shut our ears to the old prophets who still speak more or less in the old tongues, using ancient words, occasionally in new ways, we shall have very little music. We are not so rich that we can do without tradition. Let him that has new ears, listen to it in a new way.

> (Kaufmann 1970, p. 31)

The integrated person model

A model is accurate when it seems to reflect real life. So for this model to seem to be accurate it must chime with most people's experiences and with contemporary theories, so that it seems intuitively to be true.

In this model of the person the mind and spirit interact constantly with the body, an idea that Ware, a theologian, describes below. Ware talks of the soul as containing the mind and the spirit.

> Spirit and matter are not mutually exclusive. On the contrary, they are interdependent; they interpenetrate and interact. When speaking, therefore, of the human person, we are not to think of the soul and the body as two separable parts which together comprise a greater whole. The soul, so far from being a part of the person, is an expression and manifestation of the totality of our human personhood, when viewed from a particular point of view. The body is likewise an expression of our total personhood, viewed from another point of view.
>
> (Ware 2002)

To Ware, the body represents and expresses the person totally, as does the mind and spirit. Similarly, Maximus, a 6th century theologian (pp. 580–662), describes the body as always moving into the soul and the soul always moving into the body forming a constant to and fro cycle (Thunberg 1995, p. 109). Because of this integration, what affects one dimension will influence the other dimensions, so that the physical can affect the spirit and the mind. Similarly the mind and the spirit can affect the body. Malinski uses her own distinct way of describing a similar model.

> rather than three overlapping circles I would suggest the analogy of a pretzel with three distinct lobes forming the whole. A bite out of any one lobe will taste the same as the other two, regardless of naming one body, one mind, and one spirit. The recipe or pattern is what defines *pretzelness*. Regardless of the lobe chosen, the taste will be the same.
>
> (Malinski 2002, p. 281)

Often the word soul is used to mean the mind and spirit together. In this book, if the word soul is used, it means the mind and spirit together.

The mind

The mind analyses the data that comes through the senses – it perceives, thinks and interprets. It is the mind that enables self-awareness and consciousness. Characteristics of the mind include imagination and the ability to direct attention to particular objects and to concentrate. Psychologists debate about the extent to which the emotions arise from the mind. The fact that trauma to the brain can cause disturbances and changes in perception in the mind is evidence that the mind is related to the body. In theology the mind is often spoken of as being part of the soul.

The spirit

The spirit is usually credited with qualities that enable connection and relationship between the various parts of a person, or between persons or between a person and a Higher Being or force outside the self. Because ideas about spirit are not scientifically verifiable, people have used different means to describe it, such as metaphors, and mediums like art and poetry. The spirit is often described as a force or energy, a fire, a vast cavern or a precious jewel. People frequently mention the spirit in everyday language and people talk of feeling inspired or dispirited. So it is evident that people associate the spirit with how they feel. The human spirit can apparently cause emotional responses and be affected by emotional responses so that it is seems to be, whilst permanent, also malleable and capable of change.

The spirit usually represents something inexplicable and mysterious about being a human being. In Hebrew, the word for spirit and breath are related (ruach) and also in Greek (pneuma); historically there has often been a connection made in the Christian and Jewish traditions between the breath of God and the spirit. Metaphors help understanding, so that even if a person doesn't believe literally that God breathed into a lump of clay the breath of life and so created Adam and filled him with a spirit which always connects the man to God, it can still be a useful way to understand how human beings have a part of them which seems to make it possible to rise above or transcend their human life and connect with something outside themselves. Many people do not believe that such a thing as a spirit exists, but they may still believe that something allows them to connect with others and with nature, which they cannot describe.

The body

The physical body is the solid and material presence of a person in the world. It is through the body that information from experiences is received, and ultimately interpreted and given meaning. In this view of the person, because the body, mind and spirit are so closely integrated, the body is also capable of being 'sacred' or spiritualised.

Gregory Palamas (1296–1359) says,

> The spiritual joy which comes from the mind into the body, is in no way corrupted by the communion with the body but transforms the body and makes it spiritual.
>
> (1983, p. 51)

There is no 'dualist' like separation between the body and soul in this view. In some thought systems the body is like a cloak that is put on and taken off. But in an integrated view of the person, the body, mind and spirit are complementary and essential to each other.

As William Blake put it, 'Man has no Body distinct from his Soul; for that called Body is a portion of Soul'. In an integrated view of the person, spirituality is embodied and the body is spiritual.

It is through the body that anything spiritual is first experienced, because it is through the body that beauty, or the fulfilment of a relationship or an affirming interaction with someone, is felt. It is the body that allows human beings to have and experience emotions which enable the appreciation of pleasure or pain. It is through the body that people know themselves to be human and become self-aware and see themselves as whole. We know who we are through our bodies and when people see us they recognise essential aspects of our self, such as our gender and culture, because of our bodies.

Thinking time

Think about how you see body, mind and spirit interacting. Think of a way of describing it that means something to you. Like Malinski's pretzel description above.

Relationships and the integrated person model

In this model, body, spirit and mind are connected in a never-ending movement, thus within the person is embedded the notion of relationship and parts encountering each other. Therefore relationship and encounter are at the core of this model of the person and the person is defined by relationship; not a static union but a communion in a dynamic moving relationship. McIntosh suggests that spirituality is innately about relationship saying that spirituality is

> a discovery of the true 'self' precisely in encountering the divine *and human* (my italics) other – who allow one neither to rest in a reassuring self-image nor to languish in the prison of a false social construction of oneself.
>
> (1998, p. 6)

This tells us that we need other people in order to be ourselves. Without others we can become misleadingly self-assured and complacent; we can't see ourselves reflected, we don't express ourselves fully, we can't compare ourselves and we can't love, and loving is a crucial aspect of how human beings relate. Human beings seem to have been made in order to be in relation with others. It is not surprising given this, that relationship and connecting features so highly in how most people describe their spirituality.

A contemporary philosopher associated with this view of the person is John Macmurray (1891–1976) who said, 'we are only people in and through our relationships' (Stern and James 2006). He is thought to have been influenced by Buber: Buber saying that there was no difference between himself and Macmurray (Stern 2006, p. 900). He believed that how you act in the world mattered more than just thinking or reflecting and that acting in relationships was crucial to being human. He summed up his thought like this: 'All meaningful knowledge is for the sake of action and all meaningful action is for the sake of friendship' (Gee 2006). Macmurray had a very direct and simple approach to talking about spirituality, 'Our human Being *is* our relations to other human beings and our value lies in the quality of these relations' (Macmurray 1995, p. 72, cited by Stern 2001).

Hay similarly (2000) defines spirituality as 'relational consciousness' and argues that in the West, spirituality was forgotten because of the rise of individualism. The revitalised view of the person is reintroducing spirituality back into public awareness but it may be that the 'new' spirituality which people now recognise is so infiltrated with notions of the individual and the needy inner self that it has forgotten that a person is a 'being in relation'. Modern spirituality can seem wholly inward, private and expressed in solitude (Hay 2000). Yet when people speak of spirituality they also speak of connection and relationships, so it seems that for spirituality to be lived out, it has to be done so relationally even though people cannot conceive it as anything but an inner part of themselves. Even those Christian contemplative monks and nuns who live isolated lives devoted to prayer are praying for the rest of the world.

Compassion

Being a person who is made up of parts in constant dynamic communion with each other could also be seen as a template for how people relate to each other in the world. To realise that you need other people and that they are essential to your own humanity evokes feelings of companionship and compassion. Compassion is not only feeling sad or sorry for the situation someone else is in, but to wish to relieve their suffering. Davies (2001) describes compassion as consisting of perceiving suffering, emotionally reacting to it and then a call to action.

> In compassion we see another's distress (cognition), we feel moved by it (affectively) and we actively seek to remedy it (volition).
>
> (Davies 2001, p. 17)

Thus compassion could be seen as one way in which relationship is enacted in the world.

Believing that other people are essential to one's own humanity, and believing that acting for someone else's good is essential to your own spiritual well-being, could mean that compassion can be seen as essential to spiritual relationships and so to spiritual care. Compassion has been called a natural part of being human.

> If a stranger in the crowd is hurt in an accident or stumbles I will be inclined to assist and will feel sympathy, while if an object is damaged my reaction is typically more neutral. The other calls out to my sympathy because of a basic solidarity grounded in our mutual recognition of each other as fellow human beings.
>
> (van Hooft 2006, p. 98)

Being aware of the other person and recognising their worth and value as a fellow being creates a rapport which is the basis of a relationship of spiritual care. This is an elemental ethical relationship which 'precedes any assessment of need' (van Hooft 2002, p. 48). The natural and automatic response in such a relationship is care and compassion. In such a fundamental and ethical relationship, the caring offered is ontological in that it is a function of simply being human and not dependent on any emotional generosity. As it is built on a desire for the welfare of the other and the wish to see them achieve their own full potential and so full humanness and full value, the nature of the relationship is fundamentally spiritual.

Unconditional love

Unconditional love is often the basis of compassion. Loving someone unconditionally means accepting them for who they are for no reason other than loving them and not to achieve any particular outcome. Shaver (2002) has the idea that as each of us grows up we construct a self-image to support us in adulthood but when we suffer threats such as illness, this self-image is gradually shown to be illusory and unstable, as it is dependent on possessions, status and other people. So this self is abandoned which creates an insecure identity, more instability and fear. A person may never have felt unconditional acceptance before, and receiving such love is inclined to make them start to accept and love themselves

(Shaver 2002). Unconditional love is not an emotional state but a state of non-judgemental acceptance which nurses shouldn't fear. Love has come to be associated with erotic love in our culture but theology distinguishes different types of love. Erotic love is about longing, possession and enjoyment, it is the love a person feels for a lover or for God, whereas agape is not love because someone is attractive, but love because it is human to love. Baelz says, 'It is a turning from oneself to the other, for the sake of the other. It is self-forgetful and self-sacrificial' (1977, p. 105). Agape stimulates compassion and compassion stimulates a call to action, to act on behalf of the other. Campbell (1984, p. 6) says that 'consistent professional care is a form of love' and it is akin to agape. It is practical love or 'skilled companionship' (Campbell 1984, p. 35); practicality which evokes the action required of compassion, not merely passive sympathy.

Such love is an antidote to some of the difficult and repugnant tasks of nursing and Miller (1997) describes how disgust is the counterpoint of love. Mothers become inured to the faeces and bodies of their offspring because of love. Miller conjectures that love gets its value because it is through love that disgust is over-come. Nurses are in a sense carrying out the tasks that a mother or loved one would and it is love and care for the welfare of another which takes nurses over the hurdle of disgust (Alave 1995). Nurses experience this when they find that one way to deal with feel-ings of disgust or horror when caring is to focus on the person in front of them and their needs. They discover that sometimes a task that they want to avoid is easier to face if they talk to the person involved first and get to know them as a person rather than simply a body in a bed. De Hennezel, a psychologist, describes an inci-dent in a hospice when the strong, handsome Dimitri, flirtatious and arrogant and now dying, is seized by a fit of vomiting, spat-tering her and his bed. The desire to call a nurse may be strong, but this is what de Hennezel does.

> The vomit is unimportant. I don't call anyone; I organise the essentials and clean up on my own. I could summon a nurse, but it's important to make Dimitri feel really loved at a moment when his mask has shattered into a thousand pieces.... I begin to clean up slowly and carefully so that it becomes a kind of rite. I think of the nurses' aides who perform these intimate

acts all day, every day, moving beyond any feelings of repugnance because the very thought of restoring someone's dignity is enough to give them all the satisfaction they need.

(De Hennezel 1998, p. 115)

Jourard, a psychologist, criticises the way nurses compete with machines to become more efficient and more impersonal without realising that what they have to offer is the opposite of what a machine can give. He says he hopes that 'nursing practitioners will soon learn that nursing is a special case of loving' (Jourard 1971, p. 207).

Thinking time

Sometimes as nurses we just want to run away from a job because it makes us cringe or feel sick. Can you think of a time you have felt like that and been able to overcome it and get on with the job because you thought about the patient involved and how they felt?

Microcosm and mediator

This way of seeing the person as a unity of parts working together is taken in various cultures and belief systems to be an image of how the world is. The person is sometimes called a microcosm or little cosmos (Scheper-Hughes and Lock 1987). This has been paraphrased as 'How goes the part, so goes the Whole'. Paracelsus, the 16th-century mystic scientist expressed the idea 'as above so below' and this same idea has come into Western philosophy and into religious thought in many different traditions. For instance, in the Koran 41.53 it is said,

One who knows the inner self knows the external world as well.
One who knows the external world knows the inner self as well.

In Christian theology a person as a microcosm is seen also to reflect the dual nature of the world, because the person contains both the spiritual and the material and so is '*imago mundi*', a Greek term which means an image of the world. Only a person exists on both levels and so a person is one 'in whom the world is summed up' (Ware 1995, p. 50). As a reflection of the cosmos, the human being also contains all the divisions, opposites and paradoxes of the cosmos. A human being is on both sides of each division. This makes it possible for a person to be a human bond or mediator, able to unite and resolve those divisions in themselves. Maximus says, a human being is

> the laboratory in which everything is concentrated and in itself naturally mediates between the extremities of each division.
>
> (Louth 1996, p. 73)

This allegorical description from one religious world view gives an image of a holistic person in a holistic cosmos. It offers the image of a mediator which is a useful way of seeing one possible role of the nurse in spiritual care, mediating the person with their body, bringing the person into unity, bridging between the individual and the institution, the person and the system, the weak and the strong, and between the land of the well and the land of the sick.

Relationships, nursing and an integrated view of the person

Modern spirituality with its emphasis on the inner self has tended to become focused on self-repair, self-development and self-nurture. The understanding of spirituality as being lived out in relationships seems to be dormant, even in nursing which is quintessentially relational. To Rowan Williams, in this way of seeing spirituality,

> the good of any other person, is likely to become a happy adjunct of my own inner arrival at a state of spiritual equilibrium and non-violence; but it is not likely to be seen as intrinsic to the very definition of my own final well-being.
>
> (1998, p. 80)

Nursing seems to have adopted a style of spiritual care which is focused on identifying the needs of the inner self and fulfilling them, for both the nurse and the patient. The spiritual well-being of nurse and patient is not dependent on having done anything for anyone else, but incidental to it. But for a profession which is about working for others, and which includes love, compassion and self-sacrifice in putting the other first (person-centred care), this seems paradoxical. The opposite of this would be to make relationships the focus of spiritual care and not incidental to it; as just a means to facilitate patients to disclose what their spiritual needs are. Nursing and midwifery practice is defined by relationship, by the constant and repeated encounter with others. Every encounter a practitioner has is an opportunity and a demand for relationship. Relationships are fundamental to spirituality; nursing can provide relationship.

Any encounter can have spiritual effects in terms of being deeply 'touched' in the depths of your being in a positive or negative way and it can be the start of an ongoing process which colours a patient's whole experience of their disease and its management. Having compassion for others is the catalyst for being able to 'touch' another person in such a way that you affect their spirituality because to act compassionately is realising and acknowledging the suffering of another, and wishing to relieve it. In this view of the person, compassion is intrinsic to spiritual care, as well as affecting the patient, it is also what makes the nurse human and complete. Compassion calls forth the role of mediator, a uniting, arbitrating, advocating force mediating a patient's feelings about their rebellious body and seeking by mediation to bring the patient back into a peaceful integration with themselves. Compassion is more than sympathy, it calls nurses to act to relieve suffering, to act to remove the barriers to good care and to act as advocates for patients (Firth-Cozens and Cornwell 2009).

The body, nursing and an integrated view of the person

Nursing seeks to be holistic, but the fact that the body is not fully acknowledged in who we are suggests dualism. Dualism, at its simplest, is about seeing a split between the body and the mind/spirit. Van Hooft suggests that if people were truly understood holistically there would not be the focus on the body that means that practitioners forget the spirit and mind (2006). Equally, this means that if nursing was truly holistic there would not be undue focus on the mind or the spirit at the expense of the body. Although the body takes centre stage in disease management, it is very much pushed to the margins in spiritual care and it has even its most basic needs neglected if the slew of complaints about poor nursing is to be believed. Van Hooft argues that implicit dualism is suggested by the way practitioners assume that the body is only operated and motivated by communication from the mind, whereas for true holism, a different understanding of the body is needed, 'which makes it impossible to think of it as just a biological machine which houses a person's fuller self' (van Hooft 2006, p. 96). This understanding would be of a body fully integrated with the emotions and the spiritual dimension such as the model described above.

Van Hooft uses the term 'being-for-others' which he borrows from Sartre to make the point that a human is only a human by virtue of being interpersonal and culturally constructed. It is in interpersonal contact and our response to and influence from others which constructs us and makes us who we are, which makes us human. This construction is only possible through the body, it is only through the body that a person is able to be interpersonal and be constructed by his culture. He uses the example of eating a meal to explain how each part of this simple action is governed by cultural influences. He reminds us that even when alone 'I am conscious of myself as a being which draws its identity from the way it might be seen and reacted to by others and from the way it addresses itself towards others' (van Hooft 2006, p. 98). So that 'being-for-others' is definitive of being human and 'being-for-others' *is situated in the body.* We are only able to be present for each other through our bodies, because our bodies enable us to be visible, audible and touchable. Caring for our own bodies and others bodies is caring for our own and others' selves. This way of seeing the body has implications for the way nurses also use their bodies and use their presence, as will be seen in the next chapter. True holism is only possible when practitioners are able to abolish the division between body and mind/spirit in their care.

Nurses and midwives know their patients through their bodies. Even in mental health, care of the body can still be a way to affect the mind (Clarke 2010) and there are many instances in life of the recognition that the mind can be affected by the body. For instance, exercise, yoga and many other health practices are known to improve mental health as does touch, as will be discussed later.

Feeling better about your body usually means feeling better about your 'self'. When something is done to the body it feels as though it happens to our selves. Our own experience tells us this, when being verbally abused can be as hurtful as a physical blow and the effect that physical or sexual abuse has on the most deep-seated experiences of selfhood tell us this also. Victims of torture suffer from the devastation to their sense of self long after the physical damage has healed. Not only does one part affect another, but we know that if one part is sick, so will the other parts be, too. 'We are all of a piece. If one part of us is altered in its function, so too will other parts be changed' (Cassell 2004, p. 48).

We identify with our bodies. It is through a body that a person acts in society, therefore the way the body performs is essential to independent autonomy as a person. Merleau-Ponty (1962, p. 37) says 'Consciousness is in the first place not a matter of "I think that", but of "I can"'. A person knows themselves by what they can do; when the body is affected by disability, it is not only felt as a loss of mobility but a loss of selfhood – an assault on who you are in the world. Because bodies are essential to survival, to experiencing the world, to experiencing spirituality and essential to selfhood, when they break and get sick, they become the enemy. The 7th-century monk, John Climacus, sums up this paradoxical relationship with our bodies like this:

> He is my helper and my enemy, my assistant and my opponent, a protector and a traitor ... I embrace him and I turn away from him. What is this mystery in me? What is the principle of this mixture of body and soul? How can I be my own friend and my own enemy?
>
> (Climacus 1982, p. 186)

Theologian Olivier Clement says that, 'In our bodies we begin to know the world from within' (Clement 1986, p. 56). Because bodies are a way of experiencing and knowing the world and are the way we experience ourselves, when they are damaged and sick it seems as if there is a disjuncture within us, and a readjustment has to be made; a bridge has to be built between the self and the new body before it can become a friend again. One of the functions that nurses can have by how they touch and care for the body of a person is in supporting the person while this re-integration takes place and while the person finds a new accommodation for what they are experiencing so that they might find a meaningful way to live. Touch can also be a powerful medium for transmitting compassion.

Clement (1986) talks about how the body and soul are so interdependent that the body, which can be seen, becomes the form of the soul which cannot be seen, so that when you see someone you are seeing the person – and it is as if you are meeting their soul. Care of the body therefore can be just as spiritual as care in relationships and care in conversations about spirituality. Care of the body can in fact include relating and talking in ways which are unique to nursing and midwifery. Spiritual care begins therefore, from the first time we see a patient and make eye contact, when we shake hands or lift onto a bed or give a glass of water.

The problem of the body in nursing

Nursing is the only profession which takes 'care' of the body, in terms of cleaning it, feeding it and managing its excretions and pains, not intermittently, but throughout the day and night. This has been called the most 'basic' care which suggests simply, easy-to-perform type of care that nurses give. Yet it is the care that is most often criticised. It can be undertaken with competence or incompetence, alacrity and good humour or grudgingly; with haste or with patience; cursorily or completely; with compassion or with coldness. The fact that this is care which lay people can perform places it in a different category to other aspects of the nurses' role which are more technical and managerial and so more highly valued in society. Body care has not been the most popular of care that nurses perform. Although many nurses say they find it rewarding and satisfying, in reality nurses have progressively moved away from care of the body by seeking more technical roles with higher status, and have persistently encouraged the least qualified staff, care assistants, to carry out body care whilst they did other things. There are other contributory factors such as the expense of employing qualified nurses and the need for nurses to seek higher pay to support their families and higher pay usually only comes with jobs away from the bedside; it is clear that many nurses are not happy with this state of affairs. However, it is also noticeable that teachers protested vociferously when teaching assistants began to take over their role but nurses, when faced with the same encroachment from care assistants, have not. In studies where nurses have been asked to say what they should do and what care assistants should do , they usually give the body care to care assistants and allocate themselves tasks like the ordering and checking of pharmacy, storing patient's property cleaning, and errands (Dewar and Macleod-Clark 1992, Chang 1995). Student nurses likewise perceive care of the body as being too 'basic' and not 'real nursing' because it is not 'technical' enough (Melia 1983), and the 'too posh to wash' debate was well-publicised in the UK media (Allan and Smith 2009). Care assistants, while claiming that what they do is important, associate more training with leaving body care behind and so moving up the status ladder (Clarke 1997, 1999).

Nursing does not exist in a vacuum and the status of the body in nursing care only reflects the situation in most societies. Douglas (2002) describes how bodily taboos reflect the boundaries in societies about what is forbidden and what is allowed, and have arisen out of attempts to impose order on disorder. Beliefs about the body being impure have existed in most societies and anthropologists usually ascribe them to the waste and secretions which leave the orifices, as this resulted in the person uncontrollably spilling over its boundaries and becoming disordered (Douglas 2002). Clearing up the messes and disorders of the body was historically performed by the lowest status, or lowest caste people in society, or those who were culturally seen as already 'unclean', which includes women because of their involvement with menstruation and childbirth. Body care is called 'dirty' work by sociologists and it is historically associated with women's work (Lawler 1991, pp. 44–52). Much of body work is 'disgusting' and those who involve themselves in tasks where touching bodies (especially old ones) and excretions risk being tainted by it, both physically and notionally by society (Alavi 1995). It is not surprising therefore that care of the body is marginalised in education and practice in favour of more technical, problem-solving, counselling, managerial and consultative aspects of care. Effectively these are talk-based roles which are clearly more highly regarded and rewarded in society than is paying careful attention to feeding and washing. Some of the lowest paid, least regarded and least represented people in the United Kingdom are the army of care assistants who care for older people. There are therefore deep-rooted and subconscious reasons as to why nurses have not associated spirituality with the body and why nursing has chosen for its role models in spiritual care the counsellors and clerics who have a much more successful and sound professional status than do nurses. Peter Short (1997, p. 8), who photographs nurses at work, talks of how nursing work is hidden from most of the public (until they are ill, and after illness all they want to do is forget). Because images of nurses in the cinema or TV are sanitised and artificial it is easy to avoid thinking about the real work that nurses do. Images of nurses soothingly caressing the foreheads of the sick or staring up at high-tech equipment and taking orders from handsome doctors create potent fictions about the work of nurses. This fictionalised account of nursing and the avoidance of the truth of what nursing is about affect even the education of nurses where students tend to be poorly prepared for the reality of agedness, nakedness, smell, vomit and excreta and are seldom given clues as to how to overcome their natural disgust (Alavi 1995, Grant et al. 2005).

Nurses and midwives are in a unique position in society, they straddle the private and public, science and art, professional labour and personal intimate care, and technical and lay care. They wrestle to reconcile their exposure and immersion in the taboos of the body, such as nakedness and discharge and the hiddenness that entails, with their public face. How do they talk about what they really do when much of it is about a part of life most well people find disgusting and don't want to be reminded about. Yet touch and personal care of the body, the professional love which is made visible because of it and all the trust and relationships that flow from it are fundamental to nursing; it is the strength of nursing and what makes it unique.

Despite the burden of history, there does seem to be some sign of change in the air. The profession has discarded the term 'basic' to describe personal care and encourages the use of the terms 'essential' and 'fundamental'. The public are appalled at the low standard of personal care they are receiving and are beginning to protest. Eventually they may begin to realise that large parts of the professional care they are paying for is not being given by professionals and they may start protesting more. If nurses and midwives can recognise the value of their own care as spiritual there could be another beginning. Adopting an embodied spirituality which values and celebrates the body could be another tool to provoke change and bring the body back into the foreground of nursing.

> **Thinking time**
>
> Have you ever felt that you couldn't talk about your job to anyone but another nurse because of the embarrassing or 'dirty' things it involves?
>
> Think about why you feel like that for a few minutes and then ask yourself what would have to happen in society for you not to feel like that.
>
> Do you think that dealing with this side of your job was given enough attention in your training?

Holism in the integrated person model

One of the claims for spirituality has been that it makes nursing more holistic by addressing a part of the person not previously covered. By addressing a central part of the person, it has been called 'a unifying force at the foundation of holistic philosophy', uniting and stabilising all the other dimensions (McSherry and Draper 1998, p. 688). Whether the current approach to spirituality is holistic is contentious and to examine how spirituality might relate to holism, it is useful to look at what holism is. Holism is not a modern invention; the ancient Greeks believed that to understand human beings it was necessary to understand nature as a whole. Marcus Aurelius (2005, pp. 121–180) in his Mediations said:

> Constantly regard the universe as one living being, having one substance and one soul; and observe how all things have reference to one perception, the perception of this one living being; and how all things act with one movement; and how all things are the co-operating causes of all things which exist.
>
> (iv, 40, p. 21)

This view of a connected and ordered universe was disturbed by Descartes whose theories of separateness and dualism had so much influence in the 17th century. It was not until the early part of the 20th century, when scientific systems became more complex that it was thought by some that analysis alone which splits things into parts was insufficient to study how parts interrelated. The South African statesman Jan Smuts developed a different perspective that he called 'holism' with the aim of advancing the study of the natural world. He defined holism as

> The tendency in nature to form wholes that are greater than the sum of the parts through creative evolution.
>
> (Smuts 1927, p. 88)

He asserted that life was not the totality of matter, but something over, above and more than all matter. Jan Smuts saw his ideas not only in terms of the physical world but also as operating in the moral and spiritual world, but he was a scientist and expressed them in scientific terms. One of the central tenets of holism is that if one separates out and studies in isolation the parts of systems that are inextricably related to each other, you are actually destroying the thing you want to study and producing a new entity, because the original part was never meant to be seen in isolation.

One of the ways in which holism has been used in health is to define the opposite of dualism and reductionism. Dualism is the recognition of a divide between the body and soul (mind and spirit). Reductionism is a scientific theory which means that a complex system can be understood by understanding how its components work. In science, reductionism is used to suggest that one subject can be understood in terms of another. So for instance biology could be understood in terms of physics, because if all matter is made of up energy and waveforms, you only need to understand that, and you understand how animals and plants live. However, biologists would argue that just understanding how the atoms of an elephant's cells work isn't going to tell you what an elephant looks like or how it lives, or what it is like to be near one, in the way that studying the whole animal will. One way in which health researchers have used this difference between holism and reductionism is, for instance, to argue that you need to ask patients about their experience of having a particular condition and not just look at their blood results if you want to understand how to care for them completely. In this integrated model of the person, because the dimensions of a person are inextricably and fully integrated, the person can more easily be understood as a whole. The spiritual dimension is not seen as separate from the rest of the person but is dealt with through and synchronous with care of the person.

Holism, nursing and the integrated person model

Boughton (1997) tells us that physical care has been emphasised to the detriment of care of the person; however, it could be suggested that judging by the criticism that nurses have been subjected to, it is not physical *care* that has dominated but rather the *management of physical disease*. This has been favoured as it represents the more technological and medical aspect of nursing. Physical care, as has been shown, is on the contrary neglected. The argument made here is that part of the reason for this neglect may lie in the fact that we have not been person-centred or holistic. Nursing is dualistic despite its claims to holism, or so believes van Hooft (2006). He says:

> While the phrase 'whole person' is frequently repeated, especially in the literature associated with nurse education, when you ask nurse educators what they mean by it, they will often answer that they mean that a client is not only a body, but something else besides, and that it is the responsibility of the nurse to care for the needs of both aspects of the client. But what is this if not dualism once again?
>
> (van Hooft 2006, p. 94)

Seeing a person as a body and 'something else besides' is dualistic and in a society which favours the mind over the body, it is the 'something else besides' that gets attention, and the fact that the 'body' is in fact a person is forgotten. This approach has had implications for spirituality where spirituality, regardless of the rhetoric about how innate and essential and definitive it is for a human, has been seen as another dimension of a person, added on, that needed addressing. This way of viewing spirituality reflects an interpretation of holism which sees it as assessing and planning for each of the parts of a person to ensure that nothing which might produce a problem is missed out; spirituality is just another part to be addressed. This is not holism, it is comprehensiveness. The original meaning of the idea of holism, that an entity is not only an accumulation of its parts but *more than* the sum of its parts and so a person cannot be understood unless you address them *as a whole, seeing each of the parts in the other parts*, seems to have been lost.

If you look at the recent literature on holism in nursing, you will see that whilst in America the term is more often associated with alternative health practices; in the United Kingdom the term is most often used to mean comprehensiveness in care. Comprehensiveness is about ensuring that when you assess someone you do so completely, considering each system of the patient. However, it is possible to be comprehensive without being holistic, without ever dealing with the whole person (Romero 2000). Comprehensiveness, while laudable for its aims of completeness, could also lead to fragmentation rather than integration, which is the particular aim of care which looks to spiritual well-being. It could even contribute towards the poor standards of care generally which are currently criticised. Roper (2002) stated that the greatest disappointment she held for the use of the Activities of Daily Living model in the United Kingdom, the most widely used model, was the lack of application of the five factors, biological, psychological, sociocultural, environmental and politico economical which should be seen as overarching principles. She said that these five factors are what made the model holistic and without including them, the assessment would be 'incomplete and flawed' (Roper 2002).

Once something is in fragments it is hard to put the pieces back together again, as Nancy Roper discovered.

Conclusion

To incorporate any new concept into an occupation, it is important to consider how the elements of the new concept intersect with the elements of the occupation. This model of a person describes a person as being a unity of body and soul, or body, mind and spirit in constant communion, dynamically encountering each other and responding continually to each other. This provides a way of describing how everything a nurse or midwife does could potentially be spiritual care. The model provides a template for being in the world, where persons are in constant communion with each other in a flow of encounter and response. How a practitioner mediates this flow between body and soul and their being with that of another being will determine how they will be able to construct the atmosphere and the relationships that flow around them. It therefore may be able to explain some of the deeper reasons to nurses, about why they should care for others, why care of the body should not be downgraded and how nursing is a spiritual activity. The importance of finding an alternative way to relate nursing back to spirituality lies in the inability of current models to fully include the relational and physical aspects of nursing, their inability to articulate what it means to be a person, and their inability to fully explain holism. The problems in nursing are too acute and too serious to spend any time and effort on initiatives that don't clearly have the ability to attend to the fundamentals of care that patients complain about. This is person-centred nursing with a 21st-century twist – a caring profession which holds the whole person at its centre, because it has incorporated the spirit of humanity at its heart.

Part II
What Can Affect Spirituality

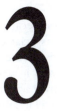
Being very young and being very old

Introduction

A person's spiritual dimension is closely related to who they are, so that how they see themselves and how they are perceived by other people is likely to affect their spirituality. Age is a major factor in how we perceive ourselves and how others perceive us. Also, different ages of life bring different meanings, values, priorities, changes and responsibilities; all these factors may change as the life cycle progresses. If spirituality is seen as a journey towards greater realisations and goals, childhood will be a time for the goal of growing identity and building security, a later point in life is a time for looking back, and gaining experiences and realisations that weren't possible earlier. Each phase of life brings its own challenges. This chapter will focus on childhood and old age.

Childhood

The spirituality of children has been a much-studied area and qualitative research with children has revealed childhood as a time of forming identity. Security in knowing who you are and having the courage to be yourself seems to be laid down in childhood. Children of a very young age seem to be aware that there is more to life that what they can see (Moriarty 2011) and this sensitivity to 'something else' grows to influence how the child relates to themselves, nature and others around them. A survey of research on children's spirituality reveals that children develop an awareness that there is something more to life than their everyday experiences which becomes an awareness of mystery including a transcendent or spiritual dimension to life and a feeling of wonder.

Hay and Nye (2006) called this a relational consciousness because the awareness of mystery and wonder was so strongly associated with relationship. Relationships the children in the study focused on were with God, the world, others and themselves and it was this sense of a relationship which added value to the ordinary or everyday world (Hay and Nye 2006), The children in Hay and Nye's research used the terminology of holiness quite naturally whether they came from a religious background or not and wondered about nature, other people and their own bodies and how these things were related to the mystery or 'something more' that they felt. Contemplating their own death was a very real experience for some children, and questions such as 'why am I here' and 'how did I get here' were frequent. Spiritual awareness and realising the importance of relationships and of other people is associated within children with forming their own identity and valuing themselves. This seems to lead to the development of a view of the world and of their place in it as well as building a path into the future with the tools they will need such as resilience, responsibility, faith and hope (Moriarty 2011).

For children and adolescents, times of sickness are filled with fears about self-image and self-esteem which are particularly acute – precisely because this is a time when identity, self-value and valuing relationships are being built. Nurses can play a part in encouraging self-value and self-esteem (Pridmore and Pridmore 2004). Nurses who work with children need to have an awareness of child development to understand how children may express the spiritual dimension in their lives at different ages (Smith and McSherry 2004). For instance, infants may show unhappiness or distress through play and drawing but later, yet still at a young age, they may want to talk about their feelings if given the opportunity. The spiritual task for infants is to be able to develop trust and they do this by having relationships of affection and security that can be depended upon. When children are uprooted from familiar surroundings and suffer pain and discomfort, trust building will be disrupted and spiritual care will be focused on trying to provide an environment of security, love and affection where there is continuity so they feel that carers can be depended upon. Physical touch is particularly important to young children and being deprived of touch and attention has been shown to be very detrimental to normal development (Autton 1989). Experiencing truth and honesty also helps to develop trust, and as far as possible, practitioners should be honest with children. Children are usually very astute in noticing changes around them and if they are not given plausible explanations they will fill in the gaps themselves with ideas that might be worse than the reality. When children are beginning to notice that there is more to life than what they can see, they need to be supported in this journey of discovery by being with people who are willing to talk about life and death without introducing firm ideas about either, allowing the child to explore as much as possible.

Nurses have to bear in mind that children may have religious views or belong to religious families; they may already have well-established prayer rituals and views about the world which they are feeling their way with, which are based on aspects of their culture or family tradition, and these should be supported so as not to create dissonance and confusion. Prayers and rituals can be sources of strength and comfort especially in times of upheaval where they can provide a familiar backdrop to the day. Children may be particularly self-conscious about asking for the time and space for prayer or to tell about fasting and feasts, so nurses need to be alert to signs of religiosity. Children should be asked about religious practices that can be continued while they are sick. However, they are more likely than adults to deny they have any, as the need to fit in and not to stand out is so powerful in children. As with anyone else, if there is any doubt, it is better to ask them or their family, rather than to take the risk that a child may be denied something very important to them.

Spiritual awareness and relational consciousness are necessary for building a strong identity and the blows that illness inflicts can disrupt this process, especially if there is the possibility of disfigurement or disability. Children and adolescents are acutely aware of appearances, and hate to stand out amongst their peers, so disfigurement is a particularly bitter blow (Stein 2008). Sister Frances Dominica, founder of Helen House, the Children's hospice emphasises the importance of shoring up self-esteem and constantly reinforcing self-value in children when they are ill. Offering choices, including them in decision making and encouraging the sharing of thoughts and feelings about the situation, all help to show children that they and their opinions are valued (Pridmore and Pridmore 2004). It is easy when faced with an assertive and grown-up-looking teenager who might know more about modern technology than most of the team around them, that they are still a developing person and therefore vulnerable. A sense of justice and morality which is still in development can lead children and young adults to have misconceived ideas about life, which might be why most studies show that children will have a tendency to blame something in themselves for an accident or disease (Pridmore and Pridmore 2004). This makes cultivating a sense of self-worth and being honest particularly important, so as to counteract the negative views the child may have of themselves and the causes of their illness.

Example

Linda was six when she started to think about God. She was sitting looking at a butterfly in the garden and started to wonder if it knew it was a butterfly and knew it was in a garden in the afternoon. That made her think about how she came to be there, in that garden and if it was planned or an accident. 'Then I started to think about God and I suddenly realised why it mattered whether you believed in God or not. I thought of the word "God" because I couldn't think of any other word to describe it. My parents weren't religious, we didn't go to church. But they listened to me when I said I had decided to believe in God. They just put up with it. It would have been terrible if anyone had laughed. When I went into hospital the nurse asked me if I said any prayers and I told her I said a prayer at night. She said that was very important and she'd tell the other nurses to pull my curtains round my bed after the lights went out, just for a couple of minutes if I wanted. I was glad, it made me feel better.'

Old age

It is contentious when old age begins. With mandatory retirement ages being abolished, the qualifying ages for the state pension in the United Kingdom and elsewhere getting higher, and the generally higher levels of fitness in the current generation of over 60s, it is likely that more people will work until their late 60s or 70s. While the term 'older person' is very unspecific, the term 'old age' suggests a more defined time when greater dependency, failing health, the often negative and uninformed attitudes of others and the nearness of death are the paramount challenges while 'oldest old' usually means those over 85. However, how these challenges are experienced is highly subjective, making definition, from a person-centred viewpoint unstable. It has become almost axiomatic to hear 50-year-olds say that they feel exactly the same as they did at 30. Research amongst the oldest old shows that even people of 85 and 90 may not 'feel' old (Nygren et al. 2007). For young people that could sound reassuring because it shows that even very old age may not be as depressing as they might have thought. On the other hand it is disconcerting because it shatters the illusion younger people harbour that the oldest old are unaware of, or indifferent to their surroundings, their frailty or the attitudes of other people. The misconceptions about how old people feel, the threats to identity, the adjustments and losses to be contended with, and the nearness to death are what influences the spiritual dimension in older people and add to the challenges that nurses have in working with the oldest old.

A Swedish study used validated inner-strength scales with 527 people over the age of 85 to find their levels of inner strength; then Nygren et al. (2007) interviewed 18 of them with high scores to explore what they thought gave them this 'inner strength'. These oldest old, with high levels of inner strength, felt they had come to a point of balance where, although they felt just the same as they always had, they also felt they were 'growing into a new garment' (Nygren et al. 2007, p. 1063). They had found a balance between realising their own strength and capacity but not being afraid to accept help from others. Accepting the way things were and not fighting against the inevitable gave inner strength, but at the same time you had to know when to put your foot down and say 'no more'. They felt connected to others and to a 'larger whole' in life but at the same time they were proud of their own life. Being close to others was important, but they were content to be alone for periods when they could reflect and put their life into perspective; connecting themselves to the past and the future. Although being able to be alone was good, being lonely was definitely to be avoided. Inner peace was essential to having inner strength and peace seemed to come from acceptance of how things had unfolded and how they were unfolding now. Many said their inner strength also came from their trust in God. As a general concept in some studies inner strength has been said to come from feeling that your life has a spiritual dimension and those with inner strength may be more able to transcend life's difficulties (Lundman et al. 2011).

Sociologists used to believe that very old people gradually become disengaged from society as society becomes disengaged from them, in order to prepare both parties for the impending death of the older generation; death being preceded by inevitable feebleness and decline. However, it is now acknowledged that many very old people stay engaged with life and remain a vibrant and essential part of their community and family into very late old age. What sociologists thought was disengagement was actually engagement in a different way to the engagement of the goal-orientated younger researchers. The supposed slide into a prolonged period of 'dying' as preparation so that death came as no surprise has also been called into question and increasingly the uncomfortable fact is admitted to, that actually many very old people are just as aggrieved and frustrated at the thought of impending death as anyone else (Howarth 1998). Like the rest of us, they may fear what accompanies death, such as loss of control and they fear the indignity of being treated as though they are just a body and not a person. Just because people are old doesn't mean they feel any differently about being ill, losing control or being ignored. They are also not immune to the vanity which deplores the loss of looks and the appearance of saggy skin (Whitaker 2010).

Believing that older people experience life differently to the rest of the population provides a familiar excuse for ageism, which displays itself in many ways such as limiting choice and abusive use of power. It also exerts itself in infantilism, treating old people like children and patronising them in subtle identity-sapping ways. Ryvicker (2009) observed how staff in nursing homes can easily erode selfhood by their attitudes and behaviours. Quiet and compliant residents can be moved, lifted, washed, fed and 'toileted' as though they were mere objects; even the language used to care for them is objectifying.

Example

We visited one nursing home to give a talk to care assistants about how they could get more training and qualifications. We needed a room to use and a senior care assistant who had already done some training and was supposedly competent in caring for older people assured us she would find a room. She then strode into a large conservatory where six or so residents sat enjoying the afternoon sun and announced loudly, 'You'll all have to go and sit somewhere else now because the staff need this room for a talk'. As the residents compliantly left the room, she smilingly offered us their vacated chairs, which we sat in with great discomfort at the thought of those we had ousted from their own living room.

Respecting likes and dislikes, respecting rights and talking to adults as adults endorses individuality and restores identity.

Especially in long-term care facilities, lack of social interaction while giving care; reluctance to disclose anything about yourself whilst expecting to know everything about a resident; talking to colleagues whilst ignoring the presence of a resident and disregarding confidentiality are all objectifying behaviours which would be less likely to happen with a younger person (Ryvicker 2009). Sometimes behaviours are well intentioned but subtly patronising, such as when Ryvicker (2009) observed care assistants dressing up residents for a fundraising beauty pageant; taking advantage of the slightly demented, eccentric and compliant natures of some residents to turn them into a spectacle. Encouraging participation was a good thing but the overall effect was dubious.

Example

At the nursing home where I work we had a talk from a nurse one day about spirituality and spiritual care. We had to think about how we could provide spiritual care for the patients with dementia. We made a list of what the aims of it would be; to help them to maintain their identity, stay connected to other people, to feel whole in themselves and to keep a connection to any spiritual or religious practices they'd had before they were ill. We decided that each resident with dementia should be allocated a nurse who had to get to know them and make a plan for their spiritual care by talking to them and their relatives about what things they did when they were well. We got together a few weeks later to talk about the plans and get ideas from each other. We thought of how we should be with them when we bathed them and fed them; we thought of planning walks; showing them pictures; reading them poems and books. Out of it we started some things like cake making on Saturday mornings and listening to some music in the evening instead of putting on the telly. We asked a local vicar to call in and do a special short service each week for some of them. It's made a difference to everyone.

If meaning is made by having a task in life and inner strength depends upon connections to inner and outer worlds, past and present, then forming relationships which respect subjectivity and personhood, and helping people to find a task to do would point towards spiritual well-being. Sharing self with others is a task that defies mobility restraints and finding ways that old people can share themselves with others in being useful and engaged would endorse subjectivity and personhood. A long life filled with experiences should be something that is shared, but nurses have to show that they are interested and even curious. Learning about someone and finding out how they have lived to that age is valuing them. Sharing their experience and wisdom about relationships, fortitude, adapting and loving with those younger is an important task of old age. This might help older people to stay engaged and stay in the flow of life as well as providing connection to a greater whole. Finding out if people have interests they can get involved in is another way of enabling engagement. Nevertheless, the value of just sitting and reflecting should not be underestimated, and forcing someone to be involved is as patronising as assuming that they don't want to be involved. Young people are usually very quick to demand recognition of the variety of difference amongst themselves but slower to acknowledge the same amongst older people who are often regarded as a homogenous group. For instance the homosexuality evident in young and middle age is less acknowledged in old age and goes almost unrecognised in nursing homes.

Thinking time

Sit quietly on your own, close your eyes and visualise yourself at 85.

How would you want people to speak to you?

Do you think this is how old people are always spoken to?

The you at 85 is the same 'you' as you are now.

Reviewing one's life seems to come naturally to older people (Nygren et al. 2007) but opportunities have to be provided for quiet reflection alone and curious questioning can help the process. Reflecting on a long life however can't always be assumed to result in peace and contentment. There may be regret, guilt, anxiety and sadness over unhealed wounds or missed opportunities. Reflection on past triumphs as well as past failures might help someone to reach the place of acceptance which seems to be essential to have the strength to go forward, whereas bitterness and regret makes you immediately old. There is a difference between growing old and being old and while growing old (growing into a new garment Nygren et al. 2007) is inevitable, being old is not. Refusing to accept ageing is like refusing to move forward, while accepting yourself as you are, at the age you are puts you always in the present time where life is (de Hennezel 2011).

For those who have religious beliefs about the need for forgiveness and believe in rituals which give absolution, these may be great sources of strength when the past is causing pain and there is no chance to resolve it. Even those who have long left religious beliefs behind may find a need for it again when the past beats at the door of memory and there seems to be no other way to find peace for past wrongs (Narayanasamy et al. 2004). Religious and cultural practices don't only provide spiritual resources and remind people about the possibility of transcending their earthly life, but also cement identities and can contribute to meaning making.

As ageing continues, awareness of the body comes more to the fore in the minds of older people and the very old still find their identity in their body and so are very much influenced by how their body is touched and cared for (Whitaker 2010). Studies increasingly show that awareness of approaching death doesn't push other concerns out of their minds and the very old crave the same attention to their personhood and identity as anyone else.

Conclusion

Different ages of life bring with them different types of development, different challenges, different joys and different sorrows. Growth and development are always possible and the threats to identity are always present. For nurses and midwives who come into contact with the young and the old at different times, the challenge is to remain aware of the delicate balances which make for spiritual well-being and to be able to change and adapt to the circumstances of each phase of life.

4 Being ill and suffering

Introduction

The experience of being ill has been described as suddenly finding yourself in another country and while some visit this other place as a tourist, some are destined to remain there, permanently apart from everyone else who live back home. This makes illness a lonely business. Michael Stein (2008), an American doctor and novelist, speaks of illness as consisting of four elements – betrayal, terror, loss and loneliness – and this provides a very helpful structure to understand the effects of illness. Each of these elements will be familiar to some degree to anyone who has suffered illness. When they coalesce and flourish they can cause debilitating effects on the very essence of what it means to be yourself in the world, impinging on relationships and tainting every waking thought. Illness may range from an inexplicable pain in a joint which hardly warrants the notice of anyone else to a nameable chronic disease like arthritis which, although commonplace, may represent a unique form of torture to the person suffering. Illness may be the frightening cancer or the startling suddenness of an accident. Illness may give you nagging, inconvenient and persistent symptoms so that you have to restrict and adapt your lifestyle in subtle but annoying ways but not be life threatening, or it may herald slow insidious decline, with the possibility of death on the horizon. We don't usually realise how much our sense of our self is based on our health until it disappears and suddenly the whole world looks different. As a person is a union of body, mind and spirit, we identify with our bodies so that no amount of telling yourself that 'it's only my body and not me' will work because when your body is sick *you* are sick. Öhman et al. (2003) found that experiencing the body as a hindrance, being alone and struggling for normality dominated the feelings of those with chronic illness they interviewed. They found that when people are chronically ill, it is as if the biography the person was writing is broken off, and how they conceived of themselves had to be reconstructed.

Betrayal and pain

People experience illness as a betrayal because it's as if they have been lulled into taking health for granted; then it is suddenly and slyly robbed from them. Until you are captured and taken to the strange country of sickness, you don't realise that your life is built on such precarious foundations. Your body has encouraged you to believe it was a friend, and then it has deceived you and become your enemy.

The accompaniment to betrayal is pain. Pain is when, without moving, eating or doing anything else, life can be unhappiness. People try to pinpoint the pain, as if they feel that if only they could isolate it and say exactly what and where it is, a fence could then be drawn around it and it could be cut off from the self, from the consciousness and it would cease to intrude on life. So patients make complex and detailed descriptions and analysis of their pain. They try to find ways to describe the indescribable. This is encouraged by doctors and nurses who all request these descriptions. It's as if those who don't have the pain can't think of anything else to say except 'tell me how it feels', 'exactly where is it again?'. When a pain is intractable and chronic, at first it feels as though, if they could only get the details of the description exactly right, the doctor would know exactly what to do to make it go away. One particular word will chime with one particular doctor and that mysterious 'aha' moment would occur. The doctor will say 'aha, I get it now, that word searing gave me the clue', or 'I see now, I hadn't realised before that it was that low on your spine, now I know what it is'. Eventually a patient may have to resign themselves to the thought that it won't go away and it has to be lived with. So modifications and adaptations to life take place, a pact is sought, a bargain made, 'if I don't move too quickly, you won't hurt me', 'I'll put up with it during the day as long as I can get a night's sleep'.

> what has impressed me over the years is how much patients *hate* their pain. There is real outrage. Pain makes the future look dismal, and it's impossible for the patient to remember when

it was bright. The body's betrayal is mystifying to patients, no matter how many times I go over plausible explanations. Whatever enlightenment I provide, the only meaning of pain for the patient is abject and unambiguous failure: one's body has not remained well. Regardless of the cause of their pain, the natural state of the betrayed patient is bitter disappointment.

(Stein 2008, p. 21)

Pain takes over so that everything else takes second place. We speak of being 'in pain', immersed in it. A person in pain loses touch with timescales. All that exists is the pain and it fills their whole reality. It feels like it will last forever. 'There is no future – the present stretches forever' (Morse et al. 1995, p. 17), as this interviewee in Morse et al.'s study describes,

You're just sitting there; again, it's the fingernail endurance. And you're just hanging on because that's all you can do, ... I can remember calling for painkillers when it's not the time and they (the nurses) will get really annoyed. [They say] 'You know you have to wait 4 hours. It's only been 2 hours. You can't have another one so don't ask again'. And a lot of times, you don't know the time span. All you know is that you're hurting and you're hurting enough that you want the hurting to stop.

(An interviewee in Morse et al. 1995, p. 17)

Pain makes you selfish and trying to block it out forces you to block out everything else so that you can become literally 'mindless' (Stein 2008, p. 26). Stein's description of Joanna's excruciating and continuous foot pain is a detailed account of the tyranny that pain holds over a life. The worse thing for Joanna was being given false hope. Doctors offered confident theories that fell to nothing followed by abandonment. It was as if doctors needed to know they could effect a cure and when that was unlikely, they lost interest. However, the person in pain can't move on; the pain is ever fresh, ever new, ever original. 'Everyone gets used to the patient's pain except the patient' (Stein 2008, p. 20).

Not knowing a reason for the pain and feeling that there may be no relief is devastating. Yet people are expected to be stoical, to keep their spirits up. Their pain puts a burden on everyone around them, because the thought that someone near you, someone you love, is in pain can be intolerable. The person in pain is aware of this and so eventually, usually just when they are at their most despairing, they realise that this is too much for others to take, and so they begin to downplay it, much to the relief of every-one around. They will maybe try a little joke about it, a touch of irony; but this doesn't represent how they really feel, it's for show; the truth is too awful to be shown to others. Patients will apol-ogise for their pain and apologise for the fact that all the efforts of those around them haven't worked. Knowing that others are disappointed rapidly turns into 'I am disappointing'. Pain makes people impatient and bad tempered and eventually people become impatient with the person in pain and the person in pain becomes even more ashamed. So that they have to try to hide away in order to avoid inflicting themselves on others. The only way they feel free is when they are alone. So the pain which was isolating because only you can feel it leads you to exclude yourself even more (Stein 2008, p. 54).

People flee from the person in pain and spiritual care for the per-son in pain is about not only exerting yourself to provide the best possible analgesia, but also in being where nobody else wants to be, alongside the patient, defying the isolation and exclusion that pain causes. When a person feels that they can no longer speak freely with those they love because the burden they are placing on them is too intolerable, then they need to be able to turn to someone else. The nurse is able to be close because they are not 'on duty' all day as friends and family are. To Stein, health pro-fessionals still have a crucial role to play, when the surgery is over and the drugs are prescribed and the pain still exists. Stein believes this strongly saying, 'A patient's capacity to carry on is critically dependent on satisfying emotional needs for understanding, love, expression, and respect' (Stein 2008, p. 12). Nurses are in a posi-tion to be alongside, listening to the pain and are able to provide physical comfort which can help to unite the intransigent body with the mind and soul again and so bringing some glimpses of wholeness back into life. If a person in chronic pain can begin to see her body as a possible source of pleasure again instead of the enemy, even if only intermittently, it may give some sense of control back as well as providing some comfort, if only tempo-rary. Nursing techniques such as bathing and massage providing comfort, pleasure and perhaps some actual pain relief also provide distraction and reinforce to people that they are valued, cared for and still included in life. Stein suggests that patients with intractable pain need to feel they can share it with someone and the best person may not be the person they are living with. People in pain need to know that they can talk about it and express exactly how it makes them feel without feeling apologetic and ashamed. Pain has to be recognised and acknowledged so that it is given a place in the world because 'If we deny its presence, we double pain's annihilating power' (Stein 2008, p. 57).

Thinking time

What is the first thing you think of when a person tells you they are in pain? What are your feelings and thoughts deep down?

Terror

With betrayal comes terror, which can be paralysing for people, just when you need your wits about you to analyse facts and make decisions about treatment, all you can feel is fear. You have woken up in a strange land and everybody around you looks familiar but suddenly a gulf exists between you. Within a half-hour of the facts of a serious diagnosis sinking in, you realise that you are a different person from the one you used to be; you are not even familiar to yourself. They are floating on the ship of health and you have fallen overboard. As much as the people in the boat want to help you, they can't be beside you. Like pain, terror takes control and it's hard to focus on anything else. Like pain, fear resists description. The person who would have said they loved change and variety suddenly faced with uncertainty and upheaval longs for their past life of boring safety. Not surprisingly thoughts can turn to life's meaning. From the midst of catastrophe and possible loss, yesterday is seen in a new perspective. Priorities are reassessed and with the realisation of the insecurity of existence may come the pressing of time and the desire for changes and a different sort of life.

Loss

Quite quickly the loss of the old life is felt, and in its wake, even with recovery may come the loss of a complete state of health, the loss of the looks and limbs you once had and even if all else seems the same, there is a loss of security. Health can no longer be forgotten about and relied upon. Illness is inherently about loss; shipwreck and wreckage accompany illness. The loss of freedom, body parts, self-image, family life, sex life and friends are some of the losses to be endured. Illness can lead to loss of work which can lead to loss of income, loss of marriage, loss of home and loss of career. There is a sense that somehow ill people become immune to these losses. This is a necessary security feature of the well, who have to do all they can to keep the thought of illness and its possible consequences at a distance. The well have to tell themselves that illness is something that happens to other people, this is how we survive living with all the insecurity of life. Each loss brings its own challenges to the psyche and the sense of who you are. Dealing with permanent visible effects like disfigurement, paralysis and amputation mean that even when you return to the country of the healthy, the shame of having been ill can't be hidden. You have visited that place that they dread. You may bring tidings of ill will.

> Richard understood that once scarred on his face, he would forever appear to be a foreigner, a traveller in the land of the healthy, or at best an expatriate. It would be obvious that he was an alien, that he'd been sick.
>
> (Stein 2008, p. 122)

Everyone knows they shouldn't avoid being with people who are suffering but everyone does, whether it is illness, disability, depression or pain. The usual reason is that we just don't know what to say. So we come into the orbit of the sufferer as little as possible. Many nurses feel that it's enough to do what's necessary but they can't give any more. It is hard to be near sadness, it can be overwhelming and we imagine that to be in these situations is always crushingly sad. Most people feel they should do something, say something, offer some relief, have some bright idea as to how things can be changed and to not be able to do any of these things means that we are constantly facing our own failure. Another reason is that to be near suffering is to be reminded of our own frailty and of what may lie around the corner for us and we would want to put off that as much as possible, even imagining it is too much. We can also feel uncomfortable because we are not suffering; we seem to be flaunting our health and vigour in front of the sufferer. Stein speaks of how he put off entering the room of one sick paraplegic young man for two months for all these reasons. 'I was afraid that if I heard his story, it would be long and sad, and it would be a long and sad process trying to console him' (Stein 2008, p. 127). When he did finally sit down and listen, he found someone with a sense of humour who was fully interested and engaged in the world and worried about everyone else's political situation, someone who didn't need consoling. This patient had transcended his bed and found a completely different kind of happiness.

It may be that when people are facing so many losses, which coalesce into losing their world and their own self, what they may need is to be brought back to themselves and their world, by being included back into life again and back into wholeness.

Ill people turn to nurses to understand and acknowledge with them honestly that many things are different and will not be the same again, but that there are also things that haven't changed and can be even better. That fun and pleasure can still be had, relationships and love are still possible, and achievements can be made. Sick people 'hover between hope and despair' (Öhman et al. 2003, p. 533) and nurses can support patients in hoping for a better future, a better tomorrow. This starts by just being willing to be with someone. It also happens by touching and holding someone so that they feel more connected to their body, by showing that they are valued and by including them in life so that the rampant sense of isolation is eroded. Therefore how nurses relate to people and how they carry out personal care is crucial to healing the spiritual hurt of illness. Nurses tend to expect patients to be well behaved, stoical, brave, positive, patient, cooperative and helpful. This is how they have to be with their friends and family all the time just in order to be able to keep people near them. When you are ill, everyone is a visitor to your country and there's always the risk that if you don't behave well, they may not come back again. When an ill person is with nurses they ought to be able to be themselves, to let out the hurt and the anger and know that they are still accepted, still lovable and still valuable.

Example

If you look around at the patients that are most popular with nurses you'll usually see that they are the patients who are talkative, co-operative, cheerful, willing to get better, co-operative, trying hard to be normal in other words. You see this whenever nurses have time to chat, these are the patients they chat to. They sit on their beds, look at their photos and magazines, ask about their family when they have time to, of course. The other patients who can't force themselves to chat because they're too unhappy, locked up in their pain, don't get nurses sitting with them and talking to them, they get to sit on their own like little islands.

Loneliness

Finding yourself in a different country to those around you, with other people who long for you to be someone else (not an ill person) is bound to make you feel lonely and loneliness is a feature of illness (Öhman et al. 2003). Loneliness arises because of the great distance that opens up between the sick person and the well who surround them. Everyone knows that you can feel lonely in the middle of a crowd. This is the kind of loneliness that sick people feel, the loneliness of not being understood because only another sick person can really put themselves in the shoes of a sick person and perhaps not even then because the nature of the things that are lost are so personal. The loneliness is made more profound by being cut off even from the self that they remembered before illness, wellness seems so far away and you are surrounded by unfamiliarity.

> he feels keenly the great expanse, the chasmal space not only between himself and visitors but between his private, inner travels and the combination of unpleasant sensations that is sickness.
>
> (Stein 2008, p. 195)

Only getting well will cure this kind of loneliness.

Suffering

Shaver (2002) explains suffering as resulting from experiences during childhood when, as we grew up, we abandoned parts of ourselves which did not fit in with living in the adult world and so constructed alternate ways to keep our personhood safe, such as status, possessions or relationships, and these help to construct a false self which can serve well during most of adulthood. However, when illness or accident chips away at these alternate ways of staying safe, our sense of ourselves is threatened because the real self comes to the surface making us feel exposed and vulnerable resulting in fear, loneliness and anxiety. Unconditional love by another person, even a professional, can help to make us feel lovable and therefore able to love and accept ourselves. Just being present with someone, listening and accepting them non-judgmentally can be therapeutic and help to reintegrate the false self, which we all have, with who they really are. In this way, illness can be therapeutic in itself because it exposes these weaknesses which although painful to experience can result in long-term healing (Shaver 2002). This can result in patients being able to transcend the situation they are in, which can bring some relief from suffering (Cassell 2004).

> Transcendence is probably the most powerful way in which one is restored to wholeness after an injury to personhood. When experienced, transcendence locates the person in a far larger landscape. The sufferer is not isolated by pain but is brought closer to a transpersonal source of meaning and to the human community that shares that meaning. Such an experience need not involve religion in any formal sense; however, in its transpersonal dimension it is deeply spiritual.
>
> (Cassell 2004, p. 43)

A second way that the disturbances of our ideas of who we are can be resolved is to find some meaning in the situation we are in, some reason or some purpose or some result that can be lived with (Cassell 2004).

Stein has found that patients want to be surrounded by competent, knowledgeable people and to share in that knowledge. They want to know that the illness was not their fault, that there was nothing they could have done about it. They don't want cheering up, but they do want to know what is left, what can be salvaged. Optimism and strength are key to what health-care professionals can provide for sick people. Patients need to depend on the strength of other people because they are weak. We are so keen to empower that sometimes we forget this fact. Sometimes sick people need to feel the energy, optimism and love of the staff around them because their own strength is not enough and they may feel defeated (Cassell 2004). This is one reason why people who may not previously have felt any need for religion may turn to it in illness. Most religions emphasise the value of the human person so infer that they may be worth keeping safe.

What people also want when they are ill is to retrieve some normality, to feel and hear and see what is familiar. Just a familiar smell or the reminder of music can affirm to someone that they are still the person they were and there is a life outside illness. Being in control and keeping on top of making all the decisions and taking responsibility for what is happening as an illness progresses is important in maintaining autonomy and personhood for many people, but it can also be exhausting (Öhman et al. 2003). These days some people will undertake detailed searches on the Internet for information in academic papers and websites about their own illness so that they can understand their predicament as well as their doctor. For some, this wresting of control out of the hands of experts is almost a matter of life or death; the life and death of one's own self.

For some people, surviving a serious illness means becoming a new person. Reynolds Price, a noted American novelist, survived a life-threatening tumour to become paralysed in a wheelchair. He gives three pieces of advice to anyone else finding themselves in a similar situation. First, accept that you are alone. Second, accept that although you will meet many people who will help you in many ways, nobody can give you the thing you want most which is your old life back. Third, accept the fact that the person you once were is dead.

> admit the third fact as soon as you can ... Have one hard cry, if the tears will come. Grieve for a decent length of time over whatever parts of your old self you know you'll miss. ... Next find your way to be somebody else, the next viable you.

He cautions that 'anyone who knew or loved you in your old life will be hard at work in the fierce endeavour to revive your old self' and this should be just as fiercely resisted (Price 1995, p. 183). Following the radiotherapy that resulted in his paralysis, Price thought that the kindest thing anyone could have done was to look him in the eye and say, 'Reynolds Price is dead. Who will you be now? Who CAN you be now? And how will you get there in double time?' (Price 1995, p. 184). Part of the nurse's endeavour in helping people through the spiritual issues they face in serious illness and disability must be in helping people to work out who they are and who they will be. If spirituality is about who we are, then spiritual care must be in doing this work.

Part of what nurses can do is to help people who are seeking a new self and new meaning to enlist the help of whatever spiritual entity they worship or respect, to seek a new way to connect with something they perceive as spiritual or to re-engage with something they knew which helped them in the past. They can reaffirm with their presence, their listening and their touch, the continuing value and aliveness of the person before them, confirming that they are still part of the living, mediating between them and the world of the healthy; building a bridge from the island of the sick to the mainland of the well.

> a marooned island of damaged men and women intent on bringing ourselves to a state of repair that would let us visit the mainland again.
>
> (Price 1995, p. 99)

Conclusion

Whatever the severity and whatever the end, illness represents misery to most people and brings with it some degree of the betrayal, terror, loss and loneliness of which Stein speaks.

> We might prefer to stay home, but sooner or later each of us is obliged, at least for a spell to spend time in that other place.
>
> (Stein 2008, p. 10)

When we return from the foreign country that is illness, it is like coming back to yourself.

5 Being religious

Introduction

It could be said that religious knowledge is practical. The feelings and ideas that people have about God are played out in practices through which people feel they learn more about God and are able to live life closer to God; religions are lived more than they are theorised about. As such, religious belief will be a big influence on a person's world view, their beliefs about their illness, their willingness and ability to get well, their decisions, and their spirituality. For some people their religious beliefs will define their spirituality because religions are embedded in spirituality. The area of religious activity and belief is so large that succinct definitions are difficult, but this chapter will explore what religion actually is, and go on to look at the myriad ways in which religious people incorporate religion into their daily life from the standpoint that it has to be taken seriously, because how nurses view religion is going to be reflected in how they care for religious people.

What is religion?

In general, ideas about religion divide into two areas. Some definitions emphasise what religion does for people and its effects and these are called functional definitions, and definitions which emphasise that religion is fundamentally about the sacred in life and what that means to religious people and these are called substantive definitions. This is an important difference for nurses because what you think religion is can affect your attitude towards people who have a religion and consequently it can affect your care of them. In nursing, authors have tended to give functional definitions of religion which have not referred to religious experts and have described religions as groups of people or institutions that exist in order to help people find meaning, comfort, a social life, community, boundaries or cultural links (Clarke 2006b). Religions can do all those things but to define a religion as only a way to have those things is to give an incomplete picture. Religions have at their core a belief in the sacred and they explain and describe a way to stay in touch with the sacred in daily life. They include narratives, myths and rituals as part of this way of life. All the other aspects of religion such as providing a community, social life, comfort and meaning are by-products of this central reason for religion which is to do with the sacred. Orsi, a professor of the history of religion, describes religion as being about 'relationships between heaven and earth' (Orsi 2005, p. 5).

> Religion is the practice of making the invisible visible, of concretizing the order of the universe, the nature of human life and its destiny, and the various dimensions and possibilities of human interiority itself, as these are understood in various cultures at different times, in order to render them visible and tangible, present to the sense in the circumstances of everyday life.
>
> (Orsi 2005, p. 73)

Thus religions enable people to structure their spirituality into concrete ways of living such as frameworks of ethics, rules, behaviours and rituals. For instance most religions will mark particular days and seasons for thinking, meditating on and generally remembering particular things like forgiveness, atonement and sacrifice. They structure giving and doing good so that these things are not left to chance and forgotten, but are woven into the fabric of life. They assign certain items as sacred so that they are remembered and venerated. They may be earthly items like churches, mosques, books, vessels and icons, or it could be people like saints who are considered to have led particularly holy lives and so are role models. The designating of some things as sacred marks a bridge between heaven and earth. These things may be positive or negative, helpful or harmful, material or mythical (Orsi 2005, Pattison 2010).

Religious people are more likely to view their religion as a way to communicate with the sacred and so nurses in particular should try to understand religious beliefs from that viewpoint if they are going to be able to understand the effect of religion on patients. People who are suffering are in need of acceptance, and spiritual care is very much about accepting people. Substantive ways of seeing religions are closer to acceptance than functional definitions because they try to see religion from the believers' standpoint. The opposite is to see religion as a crutch, as a way to provide for social needs, a cultural habit or the result of weakness in some people. Today, scholars of religion usually combine functionalist ideas with an appreciation of the *meaning* of religion to adherents 'taking it seriously' without reducing it (Turner 1991, p. 244).

Intrinsic and extrinsic religion

Allport in 1967 developed scales to measure how people are orientated to their religion. Anyone who is a member of a religion can be scored on two separate scales. The intrinsic scale measures religious commitment and the extent to which a person sees their religion as an end in itself; how much they live out their religion in a committed and dedicated fashion; how integrated it is in their life and how their religious commitment informs the meaning they believe life has. The extrinsic scale measures how much people use their religion as a means to an end and as something separate to other things in their life. High levels of extrinsic religion denote a less mature approach to religion, and the tendency to use it predominantly for comfort and security (Donahue, M.J. 1985). Later, the Quest measure was introduced which measures the extent to which someone understands that their religion will not give them clear-cut answers and accepts that they may never know the truth, but they are interested in asking the questions (Batson and Schoenrade 1991).

Scales such as these are a reminder that people approach religion in different ways and possibly also move in and out of those ways, which emphasises the importance of getting to know from someone what their religion means to them rather than just asking their religion. Religion can be the integrating factor in life, a motivation for living, the core of identity and the window through which life is viewed and interpreted (Fowler 2009). Through this window ethical standpoints will be worked out so that for many religious people it is not possible to separate their ethics from their religion.

For others, their religion is incidental to their life, and may not have the same influence on decision making and meaning making.

Religions are not all the same

Religions are not generic, while they have similarities they each embody the experience of a particular group of people, from a particular part of the world, of life and of their view of the sacred. Religions also evolve and change over time and adapt to new circumstances. Religions are often treated as though they are all the same:

> One of the most common misconceptions about the world's religions is that they plumb the same depths, ask the same questions. They do not.
>
> (Prothero 2011, p. 24)

Religions may start from the same point but they each have an overarching outlook that makes them distinct from other religions; they could be seen as each posing a particular problem or question (for instance why do we sin?), offering a solution (we can be saved), providing some techniques to do (prayer, faith and good works), and give examples to follow (like saints) (Prothero 2011).

Also, within religions there isn't one uniform set of beliefs. This is natural when you consider their centuries of history and their reach over many countries and cultures and the variety of types of personality they accommodate. Most religions exist along a spectrum of belief from orthodox and conservative to liberal and progressive. People may have beliefs which fall well outside their religion and may not be aware that their beliefs contradict the beliefs of the religion they hold.

Similarly, there is a common assertion that all religions are paths to the same God but this has to be tempered with the understanding that each religion imagines God in its own way (Prothero 2011). The God a Hindu imagines is very different to the God that a Christian might imagine. For someone to sum up the array of religions by saying that 'they are all the same really' is the opposite of 'valuing difference', which nurses are called upon to do (Nursing and Midwifery Council 2010).

Thinking time

Think for a few minutes about your own beliefs about the world. Do any of them stem from a religion?

Think of each of the patients you currently have in your care, can you say whether each of the people you have in your care is religious in any way?

If they say they have a religion, do you know how important it is to them?

Could you say what the main beliefs are of the religions you come across amongst your patients?

The incidence of religious belief

The 2011 UK Census (Office of National Statistics) reveals that although numbers are falling, Christianity remains the largest religion in England and Wales with Muslims being the next biggest group having increased in the last ten years. The number of people who say they have no religion is now a quarter of the population (Table 5.1). Overall national figures for other religions were not available at the time of writing. It should be noted that the census question about religion was the only voluntary question and 7.2 per cent of people did not answer it.

Although, from these figures, Christian belief seems robust, a very much smaller number of people actually go to church weekly or even once a month. Tear Fund (2007) estimated that about 7.6 million UK adults attend at least monthly and 4.9 million weekly. Twenty-two per cent of London and 45 per cent of Northern Ireland go to church.

Table 5.1   2011 United Kingdom census figures about religious belonging

	2001		2011	
	Number (million)	Percentage	Number (million)	Percentage
Christian	42.1	71.6	33.2	59.3
Muslim	1.6	2.7	2.7	4.8
No religion	13.6	23.2	14.1	25.0

Vicarious religion is the term given to this phenomenon where attachment to religion is still robust, although not demonstrated in the ways in which it had been in the past. Instead the many who don't outwardly practice their religion depend on the few who do (Davie 2007). In the 1960s sociologists believed that the world was becoming more secular and religions would die out. However, they have had to revise their views (Stark 1999) because some religions are thriving. The picture is mixed because people engage with religion in many diverse ways especially in 21st-century Britain. Sociologists have to adjust to exploring religion in a much more nuanced way to account for all the contradictions. In some religions people seem not to accept the authority of religious leaders and their edicts as readily as they once did, but they are just as devoted to the religion itself. Whilst globally the Moslem religion is decreasing in numbers, in some countries it is increasing in numbers and in influence. Whilst numbers in Anglican churches on Sundays are declining, the same church may be just as much a focus of rural community life as ever. Whilst attendance at Roman Catholic masses in some places is decreasing, Evangelical churches worldwide are thriving. Many people are involved in their local church, mosque or synagogue or temple, but they don't go to formal services. Attending church is no longer the social obligation it was so that those in church are there out of choice. Today people choose their own way to engage with their faith, which may not include church or mosque at all; there are many devout Christians who never go to church. In religions that are more closely tied to culture and especially to immigrant culture, Moslems and Sikhs for instance, the mosque or temple may be a focal point for communities and families whereas in Christianity, this way of 'doing religion' is declining. However, while religion and culture are closely intertwined, it can't be assumed from knowing a person's culture that you know their religion. In India, for instance, there are large numbers of Hindus, Moslems, Christians and Buddhists.

With so much diversity in the way people engage with religion and so much diversity within religions, quick fact lists about religion are not going to be able to adequately sum up each one. Nevertheless having a comprehensive and theologically accurate guide book about religions can be useful to have. Whilst it is unrealistic and even dangerous for practitioners to try to become experts in any religion, when you frequently come across patients of a particular religion, it makes sense to build up some knowledge about it.

Worship and belief

Within the worldview of a religion many things take on different meanings and qualities; for instance in Christianity, the saints are not only people to be venerated in churches but are also called on in daily life, to intercede in decisions and problems. Illness and pain may become something to be suffered for the sake of finding detachment from the world and bringing you closer to the God you worship. For devout Roman Catholics, Mary may be a real presence in relationships. This way of viewing the world as a religious reality is not instead of the concrete reality of modern life but as well as and lived alongside the concrete reality, and the ways that these realities exist side by side are the result of cultural and personal experience (Orsi 2005, p. 60). Religious people may feel that they are surrounded by the saints and other holy figures or be influenced and helped by angels. They may also bring the sacred into the material world and make the material world sacred by the use of objects, sounds and pictures. They may use dietary rules to sanctify their daily life by following fasts or feasts or make particular days holy by commemorating saints, martyrs or events. Religious rituals are also used to mark particular holy days and to make contact with the sacred in a very direct way.

Religious objects

Religions and individuals differ in their attitude to holy objects. Many Buddhist, Hindu and Eastern Orthodox Christian homes will have shrines where holy pictures and statues are the focus of daily worship and prayer and when patients expect to be in hospital or a care home for some time they may wish to have a shrine with them in their room. Shrines, like any holy place, provide a focus for prayer and a daily reminder of the reality of God or Buddha which provides a counterbalance to the hectic chaos of family life. Most religions have holy books and Moslems may use prayer mats. Many Christians, especially Roman Catholics, have tiny medals, holy pictures, icons, holy water or simple stones, which may be given to patients by family and friends and brought back from holy sites in far off countries as gestures of kindness and to reassure the sick that they are being watched over. Or they may have objects which have been held dear in living rooms for many years. Christian saints have usually been made saints because they performed some miracle, so why not ask them to perform the same miracle for you. These objects may sit on locker tops, be attached to bed heads or pinned to degrading hospital gowns and wherever they are, they transform the space they are in. They not only personalise it and provide a link to home as any photo or ornament might do, but they also suggest that there might be another reality where someone is watching over you. Holy things alter relationships and expectations and add a new dimension, a glimpse of another reality which transcends the place and circumstances you are in and perhaps each time you glance at it, or if you look at it in prayer, it may be able to carry you with it into that other world so that you too can transcend the place you are in. Knowing that the place you are in is not all that there is can also give confidence to do what you might not do otherwise.

> In the company of the Virgin Mary, men and women have found the voice to challenge their doctors, to live with or against distressing diagnoses, and to act upon the alien, disorientating, impersonal space of the modern hospital in such a way as to make it more comfortable for themselves.
>
> (Orsi 2005, p. 50)

Eastern Orthodoxy is the third-largest Christian denomination after Catholicism and Protestantism and with emigration it has spread from its usual bases of Russia, Eastern Europe, Greece and the Mediterranean over the last 100 years so that it now exists in most parts of the world. Eastern Orthodox Christians use icons, which are holy pictures in their prayer and these are crucial to the theology of this type of Christianity. Like other holy objects these are not worshipped in themselves but they point to another reality or an inspiring and holy person who is called upon in worship.

All these kinds of objects should be treated with respect by practitioners and handled carefully. Acknowledging this aspect of a person's life denotes accepting this belief, and not being disparaging or careless with objects of veneration. People derive so much value from their religion when they are sick that it makes sense to encourage these kinds of practices. It supports people to help them to stay linked to whatever gives them their spiritual strength and to help them to remember their life outside their illness. Religion is part of identity and showing an interest and curiosity in what is helping people to cope and to transcend their daily life is compassionate caring.

Ritual

> Religious rituals, with their movements, smells, sounds, and things, are privileged sites for rendering religious worlds present in the movements of bodies in space and time as well.
>
> (Orsi 2005, p. 74)

As Orsi explains, rituals are not just to be observed but they are also about participation. Rituals allow people to become involved in the sacred by their movements and prayers. Rituals bring the sacred into life by designating a place and time for contacting and communicating with the sacred. Ritual provides a context for remembering and celebrating dimensions of humanity like love and charity and they commemorate certain events and lives. As Orsi says in the quote above, they make 'religious worlds present', in current space and time and bodies, they bring the believer into contact with something mysterious which seems essential. The believer goes to church because he knows, by faith, that, as Dostoevsky in the Brothers Karamazov says, 'what grows lives and is alive only through the feeling of its contact with other mysterious worlds'. The religious person is not merely interested in worship in the way that academics and tourists are but instead

> he knows...that this other reality makes life itself worth living, for everything proceeds to it, everything is referred to it, everything is to be judged by it.
>
> (Schmemann 1987, p. 47)

The importance of ritual and the amount of ritual used varies between religions and between people. The repetition and ritual of religious services can provide continuity and an undemanding and accepting place to be when the rest of the world looks shaky. The church ritual is just one aspect of ritual, rituals can take place anywhere – in the home or at the bedside when a person asks for confession and absolution from their sins or a house is blessed. Religions have blessings for journeys for new jobs, for new homes and special prayers for sickness, dying or bereavement. Very few of these rituals can only be said by a priest and many rituals can be led by lay people. In the Jewish religion, prayers are said on the Sabbath day each week usually led by a woman in the household. Some rituals are connected to sacraments which are major rituals where believers feel that God's grace enters into the world to sanctify a particular act, such as marriage or baptism or, in the Christian Church, Holy Communion. As one writer says of a Christian service to celebrate the birth of the Mother of Christ, 'Timelessness and reality meet in a sphere beyond the comprehension of day-to-day-logic' (Mother Thekla 1997).

Prayer

I'd lie alone in my bed in the dark and sense the presence, just to the right in my mind's eye, of a patient listener behind a screen. . . . I never asked myself who it was, from the gallery of possible hearers; and I kept my eyes from ever looking towards the shape head-on. It-he, she or whatever-never spoke a sound but only heard me out as I worked at uncovering my minimal needs and feasible hopes. I never asked it point-blank, for answers-not yet anyhow. It's reliable presence seemed only to say that I had somehow to build my life on radical uncertainty, knowing only that I was heard by something more that the loyal but powerless humans near me.

(Price 1995, p. 54)

When Reynolds Price had cancer, his daily beseeching prayer was where he poured out his hopes and fears. Prayer is used by people of religion and people outside religions to question, plead, complain, thank, cajole and remonstrate with whatever they see as God, or a higher power or energy. Prayer may be momentary or last for hours, it can be communal or alone, it can be using your own words or words set out in a book, or it could be in silence. Prayer can be demanding, questioning, angry, joyful, contemplative or desperate. Prayer provides a means of expressing feelings, thoughts, hopes and fears. Prayer holds a special place in religion at times of sickness as it is often seen as something people experience as healing in itself and some patients may use prayer to ask for healing. This is not necessarily physical healing but could be a holistic healing that brings peace, acceptance and courage to face whatever comes, whether it is cure or death (Clarke 2011).

Fasts and feasts

Because religions are about bringing the sacred into the everyday world, it is natural that ordinary things like eating and drinking and even the calendar itself become bound in sacredness. In most religions there are days and seasons designated to commemorate people or events such as Easter for Christians, Eid al-Fitr for Moslems and Hanukkah for Jewish people. For people in some religions the calendar is filled with celebrations and commemorations almost every day, so that it is as if life itself is sanctified and every day there is a reason to remember your relationship with God. Some special times bring with them feasts and some bring fasts. Eating is so fundamental to human existence that it is hardly surprising that it has become touched by sanctity in this way. Many religions have designated particular days, weeks and seasons for fasting which means not eating at all for certain days or parts of the day or restricting the type of food you eat. People do this for a number of reasons; for instance, feeling hungry and deciding to subject yourself to rules for a short time can remind you of the commitment you have made to God. It teaches self-discipline and reminds you that you shouldn't let your appetites get out of control. Another reason is that not being weighted down with heavy food often makes it easier to pray and meditate. It also helps to remind you that there are people in the world who don't have enough food. Yet another reason is that it is a sacrifice which a person who worships God might want to make, to show how committed they are. In most religions, periods of fasting bring together families and communities and is accompanied by other rituals and prayers. It is often associated with extra charity to others and periods of fasting are often joyful times. Fasts are often followed by feasts and celebrations where special, traditional food is eaten and there are usually religious services held. Each religion will commemorate and celebrate, fast and feast in accordance with the events and beliefs which are important within their own world view and history. Religions that include fasts are always tolerant of illness, age and weakness and do not usually recommend that people should be pushing themselves to fast beyond what is safe. A nurse who knows something about fasting and its importance can help to guide people about how they can fast safely and so incorporate the reality of their illness with the value of their faith.

Death

Within a religious mindset, death may not be final. Religious belief influences how the border between death and life is constructed. There are many beliefs surrounding death and the afterlife and many rituals and prayers have grown over the centuries to ease the transition from life to death for both the dying and those left behind. Notions about death often include ideas about judgment and retribution so that death is seen as a time to review past life; people may believe that what happens to you after death will depend on how you have lived your life. Consequently the time immediately before death may be seen as a time of preparation when people may want to make their peace with family or God. Some religions offer rituals of preparation and forgiveness such as anointing and blessing with oil. At the end of life, there are often important rituals associated with the moment of death, the preparation of the body after death and the timing of burial (Department of Health 2009).

Religious beliefs and illness

Religious beliefs can influence how someone will interpret the meaning of their illness and religious people may struggle to make sense of their illness in the light of their belief system. People may decide that their illness is a challenge for them to overcome and that it has some value in helping their own spiritual growth. A number of studies have found that seeing the illness as a valuable challenge leads to some improvement in psychological well-being

(Taylor 2011). However, religious belief in a small number of people (most studies estimate 10 per cent or less) can also lead to the feeling that the illness is a punishment from God. A very small number of people may believe that the devil has caused their illness (Taylor 2011).

A large number of studies have explored how religious belief affects the way in which people cope with their illness and have found positive and negative effects, although the positive effects are far more common than the negative. Many studies have shown that religion can help people to find a meaning in their illness, gain control in their lives, achieve some comfort and closeness to God or others and to experience transformative spiritual experiences (Taylor 2011). The negative effects of religion on the ability to cope with illness are to do with feelings of being punished, abandoned and struggling with doubt in their beliefs.

Religious beliefs can also affect the decision making associated with illness. As has been stated earlier, religious beliefs are often the lens through which ethical decisions are pondered. Religion may affect decisions at the start of life in respect of the type of contraception chosen, and whether abortion, fertility treatment or genetic testing is acceptable (Department of Health 2009, Taylor 2011). During treatment, religious beliefs can affect decisions about drugs because some drugs are based on alcohol, porcine products and gelatine, which may be prohibited in Islam and Judaism. Oral non-kosher medication can be problematic for Jewish people and blood products are prohibited for Jehovah Witnesses (Department of Health 2009). Towards the end of life, religious beliefs may affect end-of-life decisions such as the amount of analgesia and sedation they want, whether they want their life to be prolonged, and the kind of interventions they would accept for themselves and their family.

Because religions are about making the ordinary everyday practices of life sacred, it should be assumed that there are religious beliefs associated with every stage of life and every major activity of life. As with any other person, respecting individuality means respecting the choices religious people have made as to how to live their life and enabling them to live out those choices. Just being able to live the life as you choose in alignment with your beliefs in itself enhances spiritual well-being so that religious people need to feel that they can pray, worship, meditate and live, as far as possible as they would if they were at home, and to be able to do it in an atmosphere of freedom and tolerance. When surrounded by people who do not share your views it can be difficult to express your wishes, and so encouragement and interest are needed. Prayer requires a space and privacy, worship and ritual may mean that you need to know where and when services are held. Help and transport may be needed to get to services. A person may find it helpful to see a priest or another religious professional to talk about their faith and how the current illness or problem is affecting it. Other ways of continuing with faith-based practices are through music, reading or talking to others of similar faiths and you can help by suggesting and facilitating all these things. Sometimes illness makes people want to return to a faith they once held and you can help the patient to make these decisions by listening supportively (as is described later) and by helping to get information about how to make contact with a former faith group.

Having some knowledge of religions will enable you to know what the opportunities are for healing in a particular faith and you could suggest that the patient thinks about the possibilities. Healing is not to do with miracle cures but it is an extension in spiritual care in that it can help a person to find wholeness and strength which may alleviate some of the spiritual and physical pain of their illness.

Conclusion

At times of illness faith may strengthen or be threatened, however within the context that it is the patients' chosen path in life and the positive health and spiritual benefits associated with religious practice; part of spiritual care should include doing everything possible to encourage and facilitate religious practice. Contemporary nursing has tended not to engage with religions and take seriously the ways in which religious belonging affects health and feelings about being ill. However, it is important for nurses to be aware of all the different ways of engaging with religion in order to be able to understand how the patient wants their religious life to be treated, as something central to their daily life or peripheral (Fowler et al. 2011).

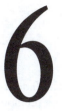

6

Having a mental illness

Introduction

It is increasingly realised that understanding the spiritual and religious outlook of a person can help in understanding how some mental health disorders begin and why they manifest as they do in a particular person. It is also becoming clear that the spiritual and religious resources a person has can help to prevent mental illness and give support in recovery. In addition, specific spiritual techniques have been co-opted into mental health care. The Twelve Step programme has long been used in alcohol addiction, and mindfulness techniques are increasingly used in psychiatry and have been recommended by National Institute for Clinical Excellence (NICE) (Royal College of Psychiatrists 2011). This chapter will look at how spirituality and religion are thought to have a positive effect on mental health and how specifically spiritual care can help in depression and psychosis.

The convergence of spirituality, religion and mental health

Sims and Cook (2009, p. 10) give a long list of reasons as to how spirituality and religion can improve mental health. They say that spirituality and religion:

1. promote a positive world view;
2. help to make sense of difficult situations;
3. give purpose and meaning;
4. discourage maladaptive coping;
5. enhance social support;
6. promote 'other directedness';
7. help to release the need for control;

8.   provide and encourage forgiveness;
9.   encourage thankfulness;
10. provide hope.

Sims and Cook (2009) draw on Koenig's review of 1,200 studies and 400 reviews to conclude that being involved in a religion seems to have positive correlations with happiness, life satisfaction, higher self-esteem, finding positive meaning, development of hope and optimism, adjusting to bereavement, having more social support and less loneliness, less depression and faster recovery when depressed, less suicide and less psychosis. It is less easy to research the effects of non-religious spirituality as there are fewer definable ways of identifying spiritual practices and beliefs. However, the consensus in mental health care seems to be that understanding a patient's beliefs and their involvement in religious and spiritual activities and encouraging and facilitating patients to continue with them should permeate all aspects of psychiatric care (Swinton 2001, Sims and Cook 2009, p. 8).

Of course, religion can also have negative effects on mental health, usually when people become excessively devoted and strict in their religious beliefs and so put themselves under stress or when they can't keep to the high standards of behaviour they have set for themselves. They may also become more judgemental when others don't meet those standards or don't have the same beliefs. However, on balance, religion is more likely to promote mental health than the opposite and it seems that people with religions may be likely to be more independent minded and confident when they feel they have God helping them in their lives and in their recovery rather than becoming the passive compliant person of the religious stereotype (Sims and Cook 2009).

Spiritual care and mental health care

Helping people to recover from mental illness, however, is not just about helping someone to marshal their own spiritual resources, nor only about drug regimens and other therapeutic interventions. The way you are with people with mental illness can also affect how patients recover and how they experience their illness. Relating to the whole person in the fullness of their whole being, accepting them and taking their thoughts, feelings and beliefs seriously is the starting point.

The treatment of those with mental health problems has a sad history and there are numerous written accounts by service users of feelings of alienation and despair engendered not by their illness but by the care and treatment they received in mental hospitals (Parkes and Gilbert 2011). Human beings have a terrible tendency to abuse their power and when given power over those with mental illness abuse seems to have been rife. Some of the lack of understanding and care accorded the mentally ill has been attributed to the artificial separation of the mind, body and spirit which has grown in psychiatry with the growth of the biomedical model. This dualistic split has not only resulted in a lack of appreciation of how spiritual and religious factors can impact mental health positively but has also contributed to the historical tendency to treat mentally ill people as less than human. Whereas reinstating the idea that the spirit of a person is ever present and holds their innate humanity might remind mental health workers of the humanity of the person before them which supersedes the image imposed on them by mental disturbance. Attitudes in mental health care have changed dramatically, at least in Western countries, in recent years with service users being given ever-increasing power in how their illness is managed so that health care is now more often a partnership. An approach which respects the personhood of individuals although their mental state is different and challenging is spiritual in that it brings all aspects of a person together to confront the practitioner with the challenge to understand and accept. Swinton (2001) explains a way of relating in mental health care within this context which he calls hermeneutical, it is about entering the 'life-world' of the person, being alongside them and trying to see the world from their point of view. It involves careful listening and attention to the details of what the patient says always allowing for the possibility that there is validity in the person's construction of their illness and delusions (Swinton 2001). This way of relating acknowledges a person's symptoms and experiences as significant and valuable pointers in interpreting and understanding their illness. The context in which feelings and thoughts occur and the way in which the person interprets them says something about their beliefs and values and has to be understood as being part of the process of healing. This is to

attend to the spiritual dimension of the person because it attends
to their being in the world and how they view themselves in life.
Thus, whilst being cognisant that interpretations and beliefs may
be faulty, they still have to be attended to and explored and discussed as part of the whole person. Recovery from mental illness
will not take place without spiritual healing which restores the
patient's wholeness (Swinton 2001). Understanding a person's
concerns from their own viewpoint brings their spiritual dimension into view. When the practitioner sees the patient as a whole
person, not as a combination of parts but as a unity, where each
of the parts interrelate with and influences the others, the meaning that a person gives to their experiences becomes essential to
understanding their illness. Mental health problems are never only
psychological or biological, but rather should be seen as human
experiences and as such are inescapably spiritual.

When people with religious faith become mentally ill and they
begin to mistrust their thoughts, religious practice can fall away,
a process unconsciously encouraged by practitioners who believe
that attending services may cause distress. In fact religious or spiritual beliefs and practices may help to put life into perspective, be
calming and reinforce the patient's self-esteem and identity. Religious liturgy can become a place of relative calm where people feel
they can be themselves, without having to participate or compete.
They may find an uncomplicated acceptance in religious services
and churches, temples and mosques which is absent elsewhere.
Sometimes the symbols and images of religion provide a stable
point of contact with the spiritual self when words fail.

Spirituality and depression

The feeling of hopelessness, despair, powerlessness, sadness, loss
of faith, loss of direction and purpose which are part of depression
suggest that depression is to do with a crisis of meaninglessness,
and is as much an existential crisis and a spiritual experience as an
illness (Swinton 2001, p. 131). Swinton (2001) used a hermeneutical phenomenological approach, to explore depression from
within his subjects' own experiences finding that they felt their
existence was without meaning and in moments when this could
be assuaged they experienced hope. What had given meaning

in the past was constantly questioned and they felt abandoned by God and everyone else. They tried to cling on to their faith because it gave them a reason to go on. They knew that they wanted human relationships but ultimately felt that these also failed. Nevertheless even in this dire situation they felt as though their depression could become a place where some positive change could begin. As Swinton puts it, using an expression from one of his own research participants, it could be a 'crucible'.

> Metal is put into a crucible and heated to extremely high temperatures, That which is impure comes to the surface and is sloughed off. That which is pure remains and is used for its proper purpose.
>
> (Swinton 2001, p. 122)

It's not unusual for mental illness to be seen as part of a spiritual journey, it can be a time of greater insight and understanding and it is often a time of creativity when writers and artists say they produce their best work. One of Swinton's participants found her depression a time of change and movement from one understanding of her spirituality to a different path. Depression affects the whole person and so it requires a holistic response.

Spirituality and psychosis

Mitchell and Roberts (2009) in a similar vein to John Swinton say that in helping people emerging from psychosis, taking the trouble to understand their delusional world and interpreting the religious and spiritual symbolism embedded in it can give an insight into how the psychosis developed and how recovery can begin. It shouldn't be overlooked that although recovery is longed for, the recovery period can also be a frightening and anxious time as people have to face the real world again and they need practitioners around them who will help them to uphold a sense of their own value and significance so that they have the courage to persevere.

Practitioners have to find a balance between acknowledging the person's psychotic world as part of them whilst at the same time realising that the person themselves has to be able to establish an identity separate from their delusions. Psychosis and spirituality are both processes that lead to the formation of identity and meaning and both may occur at the same time. Psychosis may be a time when a chink opens in our armour which leads to envisioning a different spiritual reality and so, as with depression, it could be a time of spiritual change and awakening and the practitioner helping a psychotic person should be alert to this. Psychosis, like depression, can be a step forward on a spiritual journey and the attitude of the practitioner and their awareness of the enmeshing of pathology and spirituality can affect how the opportunity for growth is explored or quashed (Mitchell and Roberts 2009).

Another way in which spirituality, religion and psychosis interact is that in someone with psychotic delusions, hallucinations and voices may take on the character and symbols of religion perhaps because of some half-buried memory or the vestiges of something read or seen; symbols and pictures of religion are everywhere around us. Religions can represent powerful forces, and when identity is threatened that power may be invoked and absorbed as a defence or may be seen as the source of an attack. Thus in delusional and psychotic illness spiritual and religious beliefs very frequently become part of the delusional world of the patient.

Conclusion

Focused, person-centred spiritual care with people with mental illness is about dealing with the whole person before you and being able to hear the person speak through their delusion and depression. In both depression and psychosis listening, caring, respecting and valuing by entering into the patients' world are spiritual acts and Swinton calls this 'spiritual care as practical wisdom' (2001, p. 175). Spiritual care in the context of mental illness is as much about humane care as in any other illness and practising all the qualities and skills spoken of in the following chapters will help mental health nurses to connect with people even through depression and psychosis.

Part III
How to Turn Spirituality into Spiritual Care

_____

7 Spiritual care in relationships

Introduction

This quote by the philosopher Levin reminds us of the power inherent in how we relate to each other:

> We are surely familiar, all of us, with the fact that our gestures of love and kindness invariably constitute an interpersonal space in which people spontaneously open up, freely reciprocating those gestures by sharing more deeply of themselves. Gestures of love and kindness bring us closer to other sentient beings; thus, through gestures of this character, we come closer to experiencing the beautiful truth of their spiritual being.
>
> (Levin 1985, p. 153)

Thus Levin helps us set the scene for an exploration of how the way we relate to each other can help us to experience them spiritually and through this, people will reciprocate and open up to us.

Goldberg (1998) gives us some clues as to how this spiritual experience can be created between two people when she analysed how the concept of spirituality was discussed in the nursing literature and found that the caring behaviours of presence, empathy, compassion, hope and love, along with transcendence, healing and meaning, are all seen as themes inherent in the concept of spirituality. She found that all these terms were allied to relationships and from this surmised that spirituality was somehow linked to seeing the person as a whole and concluded that spiritual care should include all of care. More recently, in a large Royal College of Nursing (RCN) survey, a high proportion of British nurses said that kindness, concern and cheerfulness were ways of giving spiritual care (McSherry and Jamieson 2011). It seems that how we relate to each cannot be distanced from what we perceive as spiritual care.

This chapter explains how spiritual care by means of developing 'connectedness' can be woven into the fabric of the relationships that nurses and midwives have with their patients and clients by means of caring, authentic, ordinary, comforting and empathetic relationships. Such connectedness is found within relationships where nurses are close to patients (Miner-Williams 2007). The chapter begins with an explanation of how 'care' relates to spiritual care with the views of patients about what they think spiritual care is, and what they think care is. How the complexities of care can be spiritual will be explored through authenticity, ordinariness and comfort.

Spiritual care begins as soon as you encounter a patient.

Spirituality and relationships

As people are integrated 'wholes' with mind, body and spirit connected, each part of the person has the potential to influence the whole person, thus each encounter has the potential to affect the spiritual well-being of that person. The aim of spiritual care is to help the patient to feel like a whole integrated individual who is able to find some balance and harmony, and ultimately, some meaning in their life. Your relationships and the way you engage with patients within each encounter has the potential to make a vital contribution to their spiritual well-being.

Relationality is one of the four fundamental aspects of human existence. Van Manen (2007) says that in researching lived experience, which is one of the most commonly used techniques for researching the experience of illness and care, there are four 'existentials' or themes which are essential to the life of all human beings. These are the *lived space* we move about in, be it our home or our experience of our personal space; the *lived body* and how it is experienced, our *lived time* and how we experience it as it moves more quickly or slowly depending on what we are doing and our *lived relations* with those 'others' whoever they are, human or divine whom we encounter. All these things influence how we feel (van Manen 1998, p. 102). Van Manen describes how it is in the experience of relating to others that a person can 'transcend' themselves because being with other people allows a person to become less self-absorbed and to see themselves from the outside as part of a greater whole. Our relationships with other people can give us glimpses of worlds outside our own. People often seek meaning and purpose in their lives through their relationships with other people and through a relationship with something or someone divine. In Chapter 2 we heard van Hooft (2006, p. 98) using the term 'being-for-others' to explain how each person lives and gets their identity from their interactions with other people. Therefore relationships are not just a medium by which people communicate with each other; it is through relationships with others that we experience who we are and become what we are and as such spiritual well-being can be affected by the quality of the relationships we have and the ways in which others relate to us.

Martin Buber, a Jewish theologian, wrote about what happens in relationships between two people encountering each other. He wrote about how the quality of a relationship can be changed and could be made into something spiritual. In each encounter you can either relate to the other person as though they are an 'it' or as though they are a 'you'. To relate to another person as 'you', as another whole person equal to yourself, you have to be open to them and have no expectations, see them unconditionally, accepting them as they are (Buber 1970). You can't have this kind of relationship with someone if you are using them for some purpose, to get something from them or see them as merely a means to an end. Buber calls this, unconditional acceptance. Human beings don't tend to encounter people in this way and Buber deplored the fact that so many of our encounters have become 'I–it' encounters as we usually move through life unconsciously, seeing each experience as a way of getting something for ourselves, concerned for our own image, self-esteem and happiness. So the way we most often relate to others is as though they were an 'it', an object that is there for our purpose. So Buber suggests that we have to deliberately *choose* to encounter someone as a 'you', it doesn't happen by accident. When we choose to relate to someone as 'you' instead of 'it', he or she is no longer 'she' or 'it' in a world of other shes or its, no longer just a dot in a world of space and time. He becomes a unity and can only be turned into a multiplicity again through a struggle to separate him into parts (p. 59). In essence it is as if you put yourself at the service of another and wait on them to respond.

Buber calls this way of relating like speaking to someone in the language 'I–you' instead of 'I–it'. He suggests that relating to someone in this way, as a whole human being, can only happen when the person doing it is using their whole being. So it only happens when you are being wholly yourself,

> The basic word I-You can only be spoken with one's whole being. The basic word I-It can never be spoken with one's whole being.
>
> (Buber 1970, p. 54)

Buber talks of how only in this kind of relating is presence real; that is, only in this way of relating, where the other is really 'You' and not 'It', is it possible to say that each 'I' is truly present for another. It is way of relating which is more mindful of the whole person and more mindful and so more supportive of their spiritual well-being than other ways of relating. Kaufmann, with Buber, calls the opposite of encountering someone, experiencing them. Kaufmann, his translator, interprets what Buber says in this way:

> God is present when I confront You. But if I look away from You, I ignore him. As long as I merely experience or use you, I deny God. But when I encounter you I encounter him.
>
> (Kaufmann 1970, p. 28)

God was in the everyday encounter for Buber. He was concerned to make the secular sacred, and to hallow the events of everyday life including every encounter. It could be argued that the person's spirit is present when I relate to someone as a 'you' and is denied when I see you as only an 'it'. To encounter someone as a 'you' is to create a spiritual encounter between you. To Buber, spirit was not only within a person, 'like the blood that circulates in you', but instead it is, 'like the air in which you breathe' (1970, p. 89). Thus it is something between two people. He said, 'It is solely by virtue of his power to relate that man is able to live in the spirit' (Buber 1970, p. 89).

Example

I'm an old lady now but in my younger days I had a boyfriend who taught me a lot about life which I've never forgotten. We would talk to each other and he would stop in angry frustration and declare 'you're not really listening to me'. 'I am, I am', I would protest. 'NO', he kept saying, 'you're not, I can see you're not, you're listening to something, but it's not ME'. What more can he want, I thought. I'm sitting here in front of him, I'm looking at him. This happened a few times, then one day I decided to work out what was going on in my head as he was talking, and really thought about *why* I was listening to him. I realised, with a shock that all my thoughts and aims were about myself. I wanted to be seen to be listening to him because it would make me look caring, but I wasn't really thinking about him or caring about him. I was thinking about how this conversation would add to our relationship, how it would add to what he thought about me, how it would make me look, how I should respond, what words I could say that would sound clever; in other words, I was actually more concerned with what I was getting, than what I was giving. So I tried to stop. I tried to clear my mind of everything except this person in front of me and what they were saying and feeling. Right away he said, 'That's it, it feels completely different now. Now, you're really listening'.

The relationships that you make with patients and the quality of your engagements with them are the most effective demonstration of 'spiritual' care.

Authenticity

Relating to someone with your whole being means being authentic which is sometimes called being genuine. Authenticity comes from being true to who you are and to do that you have to know something about yourself, your own values and beliefs; you have to have some insight into yourself. Being true to yourself sometimes means being prepared not to follow the crowd. Authenticity is usually the more difficult option as it can be uncomfortable to disagree with others and to stand out in a crowd. It also involves being self-critical and honest with yourself about your strengths and weaknesses. There are many areas of professional life where authenticity is important, for instance you need to be able to recognise your strengths and weaknesses to be able to see when you are about to do something that you're not really competent to do and to get help or advice. You need to be able to be honest about your own abilities to know when to refer a patient to another professional; this is essential in order to protect patients and to be accountable (NMC 2008). You may believe strongly that patients should be listened to and have the right to decide their treatment, but to live up to this and be an advocate on behalf (NMC 2008) of a patient when it involves facing opposition from authority, from managers, doctors or your own colleagues is tough. Standing up for what you believe in, or standing up for someone else who is vulnerable, takes courage but this is part of what being authentic means. Learning how to use reflection can help you to clarify your values, motivations and beliefs so that what is most important in any given situation is clearer.

Other people see a nurse as authentic and genuine when they can see that they behave in accordance with their beliefs, and this gives patients confidence that they can trust such a person to stand up for them (Starr 2008). Patients feel more empowered if they can trust their nurses and they feel more trusting of nurses who they perceive as being more authentic. These nurses were more likely to admit when they didn't know something, and, as one patient said, 'she's not trying to bluff her way through it. She's honest to me' (Falk-Rafael 2001). If you admit that you don't know everything, you have to also admit that you can never completely know any other person, which means that you can't form opinions and make judgements about people, or see them as stereotypes and still be acting honestly. Human beings tend to form opinions about someone as soon as they even hear their voice, but to deal authentically with someone means to be open to any possibilities.

Thinking time

The next time you are at work, try to be conscious of how soon it is after you meet someone, that you form an opinion or make a judgement about them.

Can you think of any times in your career when you think you should have spoken up on behalf of a patient but didn't? How did this make you feel?

Being yourself and being humane

To avoid treating a person as an 'it' and to treat them instead as 'you' means not treating them as an object but as a subject instead. This is not new to nursing but it's an idea that has become a little submerged as nursing has become more rational and mechanised because the language of rationalism is process and outcome. Therefore people become reduced to objects that are acted upon and relationships and the behaviours that happen within them become part of theories applied to people and situations as ways to achieve outcomes. McKenzie (2002, p. 26) argues that this focus on theorising, applied to mental health, means that the patient can only be viewed through the lens of this or that theory and consequently is reduced to an object, from being a whole person and a subject; the nurse's vision is clouded by interpreting and rationalising what they see rather than relating authentically. This may be the reason for the paradox of the increasing rhetoric and theorising within nursing and midwifery about 'person centred', 'non-discriminatory', 'dignity' enhancing ideals where nurses 'respect individual rights' and 'meet individual needs', whereas practitioners are increasingly criticised by service users for being inhuman and lacking in compassion (Patterson 2011a and 2011b, The Patients Association 2011).

As Buber argues, to address a person as a whole and to see them in the entirety of their being, you have to approach them with your whole being. McKenzie puts it like this:

> Regarding the patient as a whole demands nothing less than the nurse acting as a whole person. The nurse who withholds parts of the self is unlikely to allow the patient to emerge as a whole person.
>
> (McKenzie 2002, p. 26)

The evidence from patient experience is that the modern nurse does not always present the face of humanity; although nurses might argue that they are more systematic, evidence-based, scientific and rational. The UK Prime Minister has recently proposed an initiative which is supported by the RCN which advises nurses that they should speak to patients at least once an hour to find out if they need anything (Cameron 2012). Just as doctors in some NHS hospitals have to prescribe water to drink because without it, nurses will not think to give patients fluids; in other hospitals drinks were out of reach, as were call bells (Care Quality Commission 2011). Responding to patients humanely implies responding to them as humans, and humans are whole and multifaceted. How does this accord with statements like this, 'I strongly believe that nurses have to . . . divide themselves from their faith in the conduct of their duties' (Pollard 2009, p. 217), from the Editor of a leading nursing journal. Faith is only one aspect of being a whole person, but this kind of statement does give an idea of the pressures which nurses face in trying to be a caring whole humane person whilst at the same time feeling forced to adopt a false persona.

Ordinariness, being and doing

Here is a quote from McKenzie again, explaining that holism is about simply being ordinary and not about trying to cover everything.

> 'The only hope for the patient to be cared for in a holistic fashion lies with the ability of the nurse to be ordinary. Holism does not involve adding things on to the patient' more signs, symptoms, labels and so on. To be truly connected one must instead strip away towards ordinariness.
>
> (McKenzie 2002, p. 27)

So what does 'being ordinary' mean? Beverley Taylor studied the way nurses and patients related by observing and interviewing them. She found that patients valued nurses who behaved in ordinary human ways and they wanted nurses to just be themselves. Being 'ordinary' and human with patients seemed to enable the nurse to transcend the barriers that professional behaviour imposes (Taylor 1994). This does not mean abandoning professional behaviour. As will be discussed later in this chapter, if you fully adopt the values of professional commitment and caring, and are educated in skilled caring, professionalism will be evident in your comportment (style and conduct) without having to leave parts of yourself at home. Taylor found that 'nursing is made therapeutic by the humanness of interpersonal encounters' (Taylor 1994, p. 4). She identified six themes from her study which characterise 'ordinariness' in nursing, such as *facilitating* things in patients, from independence and confidence to trust. Nurses practice a sense of *fair play* in knowing what is reasonable to accept, using 'straight talking' and tolerating other people's idiosyncrasies, faults and moods. Nurses use *familiarity* which refers to the bond of similarity which enables nurses and patients to relate to each other as persons, with empathy; this included being genuine and so really listening to patients. Ordinariness includes the concept of *family* and home, accepting the importance of family, and having a sense of home, and so trying to make the atmosphere of care homely. Taylor observed a sense of *fun*, laughter, jokiness and humour in the nurses that patients responded positively to; humour helped to relieve anxiety and bridge the gap between nurse and patient. *Friendship*, or connectedness, expresses the quality of chatting and enjoying each other's company with affection, in the nurse–patient relationship and getting to know something about each other.

Nursing can be very anxiety provoking, especially for students and novices and when you are learning, it is natural to adopt roles and personas. However, this has to be balanced with authenticity if real relationships are to develop and if patients are to be treated as whole people. Price (1995) speaks of this balance when he talks of a physiotherapist whom he encountered during his illness:

> With never a trace of complacency, she quietly proved that a thoroughly skilled medical practitioner can give a patient constant human sympathy, frequent warm laughter and realistic caution without surrendering her own perspective and self-possession.
>
> (Price 1995, p. 38)

Being yourself and being whole as a nurse has been discouraged (Pollard 2009) because it seems to contradict being 'a professional' and because it might lead nurses to become too involved with patients. Thus a way of working has evolved which has tended to keep patients at a distance. (This issue of how to be yourself and not lead yourself into harm will be discussed later.)

Once emotions and relationships tend to become increasing described in objective mechanistic language, and once they become 'technologised' like this, they change. Empathy can be 'performed' by rehearsing the right words to say so that it is no longer authentic, and touching someone's arm can be 'performed' according to instructions in a procedure book so that it no longer makes a connection (McKenzie 2002). When learning to do something which is unfamiliar it might be useful to rehearse the words and gestures until they become natural. However, teaching techniques through procedures as though they were an end in themselves without emphasising that the point is to be able to leave the techniques behind and be yourself has led nursing to a point where for all our apparent techniques and theories, nurses are accused of being inhuman.

The tendency for care to be interpreted only in terms of problems, procedures and goals has tended to polarise the nurse and the patient. Nurses are either 'dispensers of help' (Taylor 1992) or producers of outcomes while patients are service users, clients or consumers of the health-care business. One of the consequences of this has been a loss of focus on the essential humanity of the nurse, and her sameness with the patient. Taylor (1992, p. 1046) asks the question: 'Do nurses and patients relate only in terms of needs and goals? Is that all they are?'

Nurses may seek to maintain the polarisation for understandable reasons to do with wanting to put illness and 'the stranger' at a distance. Nursing has developed from the revolutionary concept of caring for strangers and not only family members or other people you have a personal interest in (Clarke 2011). But the stranger can be threatening and not as clean, nice, good, or generally acceptable as your own family. Examples of this can be seen in the reluctance of nurses to use the same toilets as patients, when they would do so in a department store, or the fact that so many nurses feel the need to wear gloves whenever they touch someone, far more than is required to meet infection control policies. Perhaps relationships based on more human terms than goals and needs, and education which emphasises the sameness of patients and nurses, might lead nurses to feel that they can see themselves more often alongside and *with* patients rather than separate and 'other'.

Sometimes this approach is called spiritual care as a way of *being* (Baldacchino 2011). In essence spiritual care is about *how you are being while you are doing*, because nurses and midwives are essentially doers. Each encounter is a time for doing and being, and each encounter is an opportunity for spiritual care. The patient's spirit is involved in every moment of their life and so can always be engaged by nurses in every moment of care. Nolan, a hospice chaplain, describes how he sees the possibility of spiritual care happening wherever people are in relationship with each other, when a professional chooses to relate, *person to person:*

> For example, a cannula can be inserted as a procedure *done-to* a patient in which the person is processed as one more object in the procedure; or it can be inserted as an act of *attending to* an other in which the person experiences themselves as valued. The difference is in the realization that the health carer is attending, not to an arm or a leg, but to a soul, the being of the person.
>
> (Nolan 2011, p. 61)

The element of *choice* and *realisation* are important in what Nolan says here; realising that you can relate to a person authentically and choosing to do so are both in the hands of the practitioner. They come about when the practitioner *chooses to care*, as opposed to merely *choosing to follow a procedure*.

Ann Bradshaw has been one of the few scholars who has argued that the ordinary care provided in caring relationships by nurses for patients in the spirit of service is what nurses should see as spiritual care. She says it should be about 'one human being responding to another with a genuine understanding, openness and warmth' (Bradshaw 1997, p. 56).

Bradshaw argues that these kinds of behaviours and feelings cannot be taught by teaching procedures but are more in the nature of qualities or character traits which are not so much taught as caught. However classroom teaching can describe and explain this kind of care; it can explore examples from real patients on video and in text of what caring that will affect the spirit of the patient looks and feels like. But it will need to be accompanied by nurses learning from patients and other nurses in practice. Working with people who are in need and having good nursing role models is most likely to provide the inspiration to bring out these behaviours, which are inherent in any human being, and to develop them.

Thinking time

Can you think of anyone you work with now who would be a good role model for 'I–you' relation? Can you see anyone you work with who always relates to patients as objects and someone who relates to patients as subject?

Caring relationships

As was discussed in Chapter 2, compassion, love and care are part of how human beings relate to each other which makes them human. It was suggested that professional care is a form of love. Love and compassion contribute to humanness and making a person feel whole and valued; and being whole and valued is part of spiritual well-being. Feeling that you are cared for increases faith and hope, and feelings of being worthwhile, as well as 'increasing his sense of identity and integrity' leading to 'inspiriting', which Jourard believes, affects the body and health (1971, p. 206).

Having explored some of the fundamentals of relating to people as persons and not objects, with authenticity, with ordinary humanity, while choosing to give the patient attention, this section will explore how these fundamentals become visible in caring relationships.

To care for someone is to make them feel valued and cherished. Gadow, a nurse philosopher, said the moral aim of caring is 'the protection and enhancement of human dignity' (1985, p. 32). Loss of dignity stems from loss of personhood when a practitioner or a system has lost sight of the fact that you are a person and not an object. The function of care is to counteract and counterbalance the mechanised way that patients are inevitably dealt with in large complex health systems, and to restore dignity to persons and 'protect them from being reduced to the moral status of objects' (Gadow 1985, p. 34). Caring can help to overcome the fragmentation which illness initiates and mechanisation and technology continue, by helping the patient to feel whole again. Macleod's (1994) study identified how surgery disrupts wholeness and nurses see themselves as helping patients to recover towards feeling 'themselves' again. In helping people to feel whole again caring can contribute to spiritual well-being.

Throughout the 1980s and 1990s the nursing profession was focused on how it was perceived by the public and as an academic discipline. To prove itself as a profession, one of the tools it adopted was an analysis of the idea of caring and how it was perceived by patients and nurses. The overall conclusion was that caring was what marked nursing out as different because although other professions were full of individuals who no doubt 'cared', one of nursing's reasons for existing was to care. What also emerged was that patients perceived care in slightly different ways to nurses. To patients, efficiency, clinical expertise and giving honest clear information seemed to denote good care at least as much as the more emotional and expressive behaviour which nurses tended to think of first (e.g. von Essen and Sjödén 1991). However, there were specific behaviours not necessarily related to efficient nursing practice which impressed patients as being caring, such as being treated as an individual. Patients were also keen to state that they could tell if someone was being inauthentic; they knew if someone was just acting kind while still seeing them as an object (Åstedt-Kürki and Haggman-Laitila 1992).

In Drew's seminal study (1986), patients said that the nurses whom they felt did not care for them were 'starchy, cold, stiff, mechanical, indifferent, bored, impatient, irritated, flip, close-minded, superior, disinterested, dismissive, insensitive and preoccupied' and 'lacking emotional warmth' (p. 41). These qualities were exemplified by behaviours such as lack of eye contact, inexpressive 'dead pan' tones of voice, using false endearments and being hurried, among others. If they experienced the kind of negative behaviour described above, they felt they were 'being a bother', 'asking more than they should', they felt stupid and insignificant, a 'nobody', 'out of place and out of line', excluded, on the outside of life. They did not have these feelings of exclusion if they were somehow able to cope with the 'anger, fear or shame' provoked in them, and then they might manage to 'maintain self-esteem' (p. 41). Whereas if they felt that energy and effort was being used for them, they felt confirmed in themselves and included. When they felt that carers liked their work and cared about what happened to them, when they were patient, undisturbed by mess and gore, and looked like they were making efforts to understand them, patients felt cared for and confirmed.

Being able to see that a nurse was enjoying their work was very important. One woman who had just given birth spoke of caring behaviour as the midwife yelling to her husband to come and see the head of her baby crowning, 'she was as excited as he was' (p. 42). When they experienced these positive qualities from nurses they felt they could make decisions for themselves and they felt they had the strength to recover. They felt 'hope, comfort, confident and assurance' (p. 42). Patients who experienced confirming behaviour felt, in the words of one patient, 'stronger as a person, that I was more in control' (p. 42), whereas excluding behaviour was exhausting and left them too stressed and tired to cope with their illness.

Drew concluded that the results of negative behaviours on patients were feelings of exclusion and depersonalisation while the positive feelings they experienced when care was good, provoked the opposite which was a feeling of being confirmed and validated as a person. Drew cites van Den Berg to explain:

> when excluded we see ourselves and our bodies as undesirable, unwanted and we cannot inhabit our bodies easily and freely as we would when we feel accepted and confirmed by others. There grows a split between mind and body, we become embarrassed, ashamed, self-conscious.
>
> (van den Berg 1955, p. 55, cited by
> Drew 1986, p. 39)

Thus care which has a depersonalising effect will impact on the whole person *including* how they feel about their body.

The idea of nursing being both an art and a science was a concept that had grown as a response to efforts to explain those aspects of nursing which didn't seem to fit into the dominant scientific paradigm. Appleton's (1993) interviews with patients and nurses suggest that the art of nursing is expressed in caring which focuses on the whole person and involves compassion for the patient as well as a willingness by nurses to get personally involved. Caring which truly expresses the art of nursing is caring which focuses on 'being with' the patient as well as doing for. It involves having a relationship with patients in which both patient and nurse flourish. Patients felt that in order for these kinds of relationships to develop, nurses had to act with empathy; they had to trust that the nurse had their best interests at heart and they had to have confidence in the nurse's knowledge and skills (Appleton 1993). This confidence allowed the patients to express themselves and feel some degree of liberation and freedom to be themselves. Nurses and patients described something akin to 'transcendent togetherness' (p. 896). They described such relationships as helping both parties to rise above the problems and woes of the illness and the everyday and to reach a new perspective such that, 'In this way, the nurse and patient relate feeling they are a part of something greater than themselves' (p. 896). The participants of this study expressed feeling that there was a 'different energy going on' which one patient talked of as spiritual. Appleton (1993, p. 897) calls this 'enspiriting' as a way of explaining what seems to be happening when a caring relationship really worked.

Comfort

For nurses who care for embodied beings, care is associated with comfort. Comfort for most nurses suggests a state of bodily comfort and nurses frequently talk about making someone comfortable but more exploration into how patients experience comfort seems to suggest that the concept could have much more far reaching connotations. Comfort is a state of being content with or able to live with a particular situation, be it a temporary ache in a leg or the news of a bad prognosis. We speak today of being 'comfortable' with an idea or a change for instance. The word comfort comes from the Latin *confortare*, which means 'to strengthen', an idea that seems to have become lost to nursing. Problems and symptoms cannot all be eradicated instantly, but people can be helped to become 'comfortable' with them and so to be strengthened in their ability to manage or overcome them. Similarly, a nurse may give 'comfort' in the form of consoling or reassuring words which can serve to strengthen resolve and may help someone to live with their situation while they muster their own spiritual reserves or it may enhance their own spiritual resources. Providing physical comfort in physical care is an essential act of spiritual care in therapeutic nursing not only as an expression of caring and compassion but also because it enables reintegration and reconnection with failing bodies (a subject which is addressed in a later chapter). Nurses can be doing all these things when they 'make you comfortable'.

> The sense of comfort and reassurance conveyed by the careful tucking-in of a blanket, turning a pillow, adjusting clothes, putting papers and handkerchiefs within easy reach; and the warm smile which says silently, 'you're all right now!; may not be noticed by another, but to the patient it all means so much. It is a silent but eloquent language between two people

brought together in a trouble shared. The patient's burden is lightened for he knows he is not completely alone.

(Pearce 1969, p. 78)

This last quote is from a book long out of print which was a standard nursing textbook of the 1950s and 1960s. It expresses some of the ordinary care which shows patients that they are valued and not alone. Ordinary care such as this connects the patient to themselves as a person and by so doing reminds them that they are still connected to life. By addressing the small needs of a person as well as the larger needs, the patient sees and experiences daily, how valuable they are. Connection to themselves and connection to their own body are lost when illness strikes and comfort could be seen as a state of some temporary adjustment or truce with the body or even as an ultimate goal of nursing (Morse et al. 1995). Bottorff studied what patients say about comfort and concluded this:

> our comfort is experienced in relation to our stance in the world-as patients overwhelmed by the pain of fatigue, exhaustion, illness. Through the experience of comfort we become connected to the world again. It is our bridge to life, to living.
>
> (Bottorff 1991, p. 250)

Thinking time
What does the word 'comfort' mean to you? Do you feel 'comfortable' in the world, with your life? How does that feel?

Conclusion

The image of the bridge reminds us of the role the nurse can play in mediating and connecting between the patient and the rest of the world, the physical body and the spiritual self, helping the patient to feel connected and whole again. What these studies tell us is something about the link between what constitutes care and comfort and what patients say they want to meet their spiritual needs (e.g. Taylor and Mamier 2005, Tanyi et al. 2006). While it's not always evident in writing about spiritual care, nurses seem to sense that being comfortable is a part of spiritual well-being (Noble and Jones 2010). It seems that care-giving offered in open, warm, human ways, with compassion, within I–you relationships that are person-centred, where the nurse is fully involved, seem to elicit feelings of value, inclusion, connection, wholeness, courage, transcendence, confidence, self-esteem, freedom, self-expression, wholeness and integration within patients, all of which are factors associated with spiritual well-being. As Evelyn Pearce said in another era,

> By her understanding a nurse can change the whole outlook of a patient in hospital from one of embarrassment and anxiety to confidence and peace.
>
> (Pearce 1969, p. 89)

Changing the outlook of a patient is a good way to describe what spiritual care can do, when it is embedded in the simple acts of care.

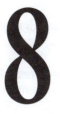

Some skills for spiritual care in relationships

Introduction

This chapter will look at the skills of spiritual care which are the skills that help nurses to make connections with patients and so help patients to feel connected within themselves and to others. This kind of care is focused on the patient and puts them at the centre of each encounter, it is a style of communicating which addresses the patient as a whole person and is empathetic and engaged. It is built on encounters which are 'I–you' in nature rather than 'I–it' It emphasises comfort and acknowledges how feelings of value, safety and respect are rooted in comfort. Here you will see how using body language, showing empathy and using your own presence can enable you to make your own self an instrument of spiritual care.

Sharing, caring and attending

As we saw in the studies discussed earlier, the qualities which patients recognised as demonstrating this kind of connected and engaged care were all demonstrated by the way nurses carried out clinical tasks, the things they said, the way they made eye contact, their positioning and their energetic tone of voice. Patients who felt confirmed and included in Drew's study said that the signs that a nurse is engaged with them and listening are that they lean towards them, they act energetically, they sit on the same level as them, they make eye contact and they appear unhurried. Patients in Drew's study said, 'I could see in her eyes that she wanted to understand what I was trying to say', 'They bent over to talk to me', 'She comes close and looks at you', 'He sits down where I can see', 'He leaned forward' (Drew 1986, p. 42), whereas patients felt excluded and depersonalised when nurses acted as though they were hurried, avoided eye contact, had a flat tone of voice and an abrupt manner of speaking (Drew 1986).

Edwards (1998) explored how touch and space are interpreted by older patients and found similarly that the position the nurse adopted was crucial:

> All patients expressed a preference for staff to sit or bend down when communicating with them, this gave them a sense of ease, was friendlier and made them feel that the staff was interested in them: whereas when staff remained standing they appeared distant, uncaring and aloof.
>
> (Edwards 1998, p. 814)

Eye contact, or 'gaze' as psychologists call it, denotes attention and intimacy while lack of gaze denotes inattention and passivity (Argyle 1988). Levels of gaze and rules about gaze vary among different cultures with, for instance, Arabic cultures using more gaze and Japanese cultures using less. In the United Kingdom, making eye contact is considered a sign of engagement and honesty and is highly prized, with lack of eye contact often being harshly judged. People usually assume that attention is waning when the eyes wander too much. People often praise the quality in others of being able to make anyone they speak to feel as though they are the only person in the room or the only person who mattered; an effect that can be achieved with eye contact. It is far better to try to make eye contact on an initial meeting and have to modify your approach later with a particular person, than to never make eye contact and risk alienating a far greater number of people. In situations of high emotion, or where people are undressed and vulnerable, constant eye contact can be intrusive so the amount of gaze has to be gauged to the situation and usually people do this naturally.

Patients appreciated it when nurses didn't act as if hurried and it is possible to feel rushed and to still act in a slow and unhurried manner. This was particularly appreciated and had a profound effect on patients in most studies. It is possible even in the smallest moment to give a person your whole attention as will be discussed later.

Wysong and Driver (2009), in interviews found that ICU patients' perceptions of skilled nursing care focused predominantly on their interpersonal rather than technical skills. These patients judged competence by friendliness, cheerfulness, compassion, being able to bond, being interested in the patient, confidence and not being rushed. Similarly Fosbinder (1994) used interviews and observations to explore how patients perceived good care and found that when patients were asked about episodes of care they focused almost entirely on how the nurse interacted with them. Fosbinder subsequently developed a theory of interpersonal competence in four parts, *translating, getting to know you, establishing trust and going the extra mile. Translating* was about keeping patients informed by giving clear information and instructions which on its own can transmit care and interest. To take the trouble to explain something in detail shows tremendous concern for a patient and it is a way to express that you value and care for someone and may come more naturally to some nurses than quietness and presence. Taking trouble to explain something, making eye contact and using touch while you do it can be an important way in itself to establish an engaged and empathic relationship. A patient in Fosbinder's study was particularly affected by a nurse kneeling on the floor besides her bed in order to get at the right level to look directly into her eyes. The second part of interpersonal competence, *getting to know you* involved the nurse sharing information about herself and using humour. One of the factors that Taylor (1992) also proposes as an essential part of ordinary nursing is the ability to use humour. Humour softens the contours of harsh reality with laughter. Sharing a joke encourages the sharing of relationship, it creates connection and a joke can very quickly move a relationship onto a deeper plane. The patients in Drew's study thought that 'their positive experiences involved caregivers who smiled and joked with them' (Drew 1986, p. 42). Taylor and Mamier (2005) found in their group of 156 cancer patients, that in terms of spiritual care, considerably more of them wanted the nurse to bring them something humorous than wanted her to listen to their spiritual concerns. Fosbinder (1994) found that nurses sharing some information about themselves and sharing a joke was central to how the relationship developed. Humour is often used to disperse embarrassment and patients value it when personal care is happening and there is potential for embarrassment. Patients felt that they got to know nurses better and they became more human if they disclosed something about themselves and it made them feel as though they belonged. *Establishing trust* happened when patients had confidence in the nurse and this came about through nurses looking efficient and doing what was promised. Trusting relationships developed when nurses were prompt in giving care and when they checked on patients when they said they would. Fosbinder and other studies (e.g. Wysong and Driver 2009) also found that patients seemed to have more trust in nurses who looked like they were enjoying their job. The final factor in developing caring relationships was in *going the extra mile* (Fosbinder 1994, p. 1089). To patients this happened when a nurse appeared to do more than she absolutely had to, when they seemed to make their care personal, and they showed real interest in the patient. As one patient said,

> One was a gem last night. She got emotional with me, she held my hand. Going by the book is good, that is the way I run my business but a gem does more, she took a moment away from being a nurse, thinking about medicine, she was compassionate. She said to me, 'if you doze off, don't worry, I'll be here'. That made me feel good. There is the little extra smile. You need a human touch. The really good nurses do more than just be 'formal'.
>
> (Fosbinder 1994, p. 1089)

Example

I'd waited all morning for Tracy to find the time to sit down and listen to me. I saw her flying around with the drug trolley and then one person after another going up to her and asking her things. I thought she'd never find the time for me, even though I told her after breakfast that I needed to have a chat. Eventually she turned up, apologised and pulled the curtains round the bed and sat down. Just that, pulling the curtains and sitting down and then looking straight at me made me feel like she was ready to listen. I know the curtains don't cut out noise but they do make a kind of statement about privacy so that was great. Well I started to tell her how I felt about going home to my son's, and no sooner had I started than that ward clerk poked her head through the curtains and said all sprightly like, 'Phone call from Mr Burke, Tracy'. I thought, well that's it then, he's a consultant, she'll go off. But she didn't! I was so shocked, she hardly took her eyes off me and said over her shoulder 'Tell him I'll ring back, I'm talking to Mrs Scott'. Well I nearly fell off the bed with surprise and I was so moved I thought I'd cry. I suppose it was all the emotion of the operation or something. I could see the ward clerk was a bit peeved and she tutted and went off. Tracy just ignored her and looked at me, and said 'now where were we'. It made me feel like I really mattered.

Empathy

At the centre of patient focused, engaged care is empathy which is about the ability to put yourself in someone else's shoes, to see the world from their point of view, and even to feel what they feel. This is possible because nurses and patients share a common humanity and nurses have experiences, feelings, memories and imagination they can draw on which have similarities to what the patient is experiencing. Nobody wants to hear someone say, 'I know exactly what you're going through' because 'exactly' or completely knowing another person is never possible and to suggest that it is devalues their own experience. Nevertheless it is possible to enter into another person's experience by using memory and imagination. This is what happens when someone who has never given birth becomes an exceptionally sensitive midwife, or when a novelist writes about a war which they have never experienced, so that a reader who has experienced it feels that the writer knows exactly how they felt as if they had been there. Sometimes this seems almost uncanny. Similarly most people have experienced a person being insensitive and un-empathetic towards them even when they have had the same problem themselves. Therefore having had exactly the same experience is neither necessary for nor a guarantee of empathy. Empathy is embedded in communication and you can express it by ordinary expressions of sympathy and pity as well as the learnt and 'professional responses' of objectively repeating and reflecting back what the patient says. An emphasis on this taught, psychotherapeutic, empathetic style has unfortunately tended to replace the ordinary human response in nursing of words of sympathy and consolation (Morse et al. 1992) which has made some nurses feel that they can't offer empathetic support unless specially trained. Caring empathetic communication is always focused on the patient, but the nurse has to be willing to engage emotionally and be willing to share in what the patient is feeling. They might respond to a patient's distress by feeling pity, sympathy and compassion and should not be shy of using consoling behaviour. These kinds of responses are spontaneous and express ordinary human caring (Morse et al. 1992). Consolation will be explored later.

Presence

'Presence' is a term used to describe when you are not only physically 'present' with someone, but you have put your whole self in their presence and at their service. 'Presence' takes place in a moment of contact when one person encounters another in an I–you relationship. When you are really present, you are making yourself completely available to another person.

You can be really present with someone in a fleeting moment or in a short conversation. Or you can be 'with' someone in a stolen few minutes of silence. Bottorff (1991) cites the philosopher Marcel (1969) on instances when someone can be physically present but not really 'present'.

> There are some people who reveal themselves as 'present'-that is to say, at our disposal-when we are in pain or need to confide in someone, while there are other people who do not give this feeling, however great is their good will. The most attentive listener may give me the impression of not being present; he gives me nothing, he cannot make room for me in himself whatever the material favours he is prepared to grant me. The truth is there is a way of listening which is a way of giving, and another way which is a way of refusing. Presence is something which reveals itself immediately and unmistakably in a look, a smile, an intonation, or a handshake.
>
> (Marcel 1969, pp. 25, 26)

You have these opportunities, like Marcel describes, to be really present with someone when you are busy performing clinical care. A woman in Bottorff's study (1991, p. 244) said this about her midwife during labour:

> I felt I was listened to through body contact and body language more so than in mutual conversation. Strange, so often the words are forgotten where a feeling or presence remains of an experience. She was there totally just for me.
>
> (Diane)

Thinking time

Have you ever been talking to someone and felt that they were not listening, not really with you at all. How did it make you feel? How does it make you feel when you know someone is giving you their whole attention? Have you ever had that experience?

When a person feels that you are really present with them they are more likely to feel secure and valued. They are less likely to feel they have to hide their feelings. It is like feeling sure that someone is on your side, looking out for you. Buber talks of how only in I–you relating can presence be real; that is, only in this way of relating, where the other is really 'You' and not 'It', is it possible to say that each 'I' is truly present for the other person. 'Only as the You becomes present does presence come into being' (Buber 1970, p. 64). Nurses are busy and to sit next to someone for long periods of time will seem impossible. But presence doesn't take time, it takes attention.

Example

Mr Ahmed lay in his bed all day watching the nurses running back and forth past the end of his bed, always busy, always something to do. It was a surgical ward, there were so many sick people, going to and from the theatre. His operation was over, he didn't have much to worry about now except his wound, his drip and his bowels, but what was that compared to these poor people. One he even saw with two big tubes coming out of his chest! But there was one little nurse who now and then when she passed, would stop for a few seconds, squeeze his toes through the bedclothes, smile, look right into his eyes and mouth the words quietly, as though they were just for him, 'are you alright?', in that moment he knew that he was the most important person in the ward for her. As long as she kept on doing that now and then he knew he was being cared for. He knew that if he said he was sick, she would stop everything and come to his side.

Although most of your time is taken up with actions, more than other professionals, you are in the position of being able to be with patients without speaking. This kind of engagement with patients, when it takes place in quietness and is not associated with activity, creates a place between two people that is full of waiting and full of endurance. You wait upon the other person to speak or not to speak, to give or not to give. You allow the moment to unfold whatever way it will and endure the wait. You endure the silence and allow the moment to just be, with both of you within it. This kind of communication turns a moment into an expanse of engagement. Sometimes words are not necessary and all you have to do is be there, but without anything else occupying your thoughts. Liehr describes how presence, whether when you are busy or just sitting, is a gift.

As one matures in nursing, it becomes increasingly clear that the unique gift a nurse has to offer is to share self by being present with another.

(Liehr 1989)

Presence can take place in any encounter where you are giving someone your whole attention, using body position, eye contact, an energetic but calm tone of voice and touch to establish rapport (Fredriksson 1999). In a particular interaction, when the patient is working through thoughts and feelings and questions about their own spiritual journey, having a hopeful and caring presence with them can be reassuring and supportive; time may pass and there is a need to be silent and not to try to force someone to move to another phase or another question. To just be with someone but to be silent and attentive and available can be a powerful experience.

Example

I felt so silly. I knew it could be a lot worse. At least they'd caught it early. But I knew it would mean that the breast would have to come off. I'd get back to work and have a reconstruction and all of that, so it would be alright. But it just felt like I had turned into someone else. Suddenly I was this sick person; I knew nothing would be the same again, I didn't recognise myself. Carol wasn't there when they told me, but she went past the end of my bed and saw me all red eyed. She said 'so they've told you then'. Then she just put down the tray she was carrying and pulled the curtains around the bed. What's she doing, I thought, there's nothing she can say that will make this better. There's nothing I want to say. She pulled up a chair and sat there. It was quiet and I thought, am I supposed to say something? But I don't want to say anything. So we both just sat there. She looked at me and touched my hand and looked at me and at my hand and I just felt this attention. She just, well..., just sat there as though we were just letting the whole thing sink in. It was weird at first, then I started to feel a bit better. It could have been 10 minutes but it was probably only a couple of minutes. I felt like she really cared about me and as though she knew how I felt. She looked kind of positive but realistic. Somehow I could begin to see how I might be able to incorporate this big change into who I was. It had to be done somehow and I had to do it. Hope came from somewhere. We didn't have to say anything. Then she gave my hand a squeeze and said we can have a talk later if you want. It was just right.

Through presence nurses can show the unconditional love and acceptance which can help someone to love and accept themselves more, which Shaver explains, is essential for dealing with the blows to the sense of selfhood which events which shake our security cause (Shaver 2002).

How do I make myself care?

Expressing caring and being really present with someone doesn't require effort to act correctly or to conjure up the correct emotions. This is because, as was discussed in Chapter 2, and as van Hooft theorises below, the whole self is present in the body and so you only have to care skilfully and carefully, with professional commitment and with attention to the patient and the task for this to be clear to patients.

> If a person is authentically present in their bodily comportment and if that person has the professional commitment appropriate to a health worker, then that bodily comportment will be an expressive presence for the other which conveys the authenticity of the health worker's care. Because our bodies are the locus of our social and cultural being, nurses do not need to be deliberate and strategic so as to express caring. They do not need to inspect their inner lives to see if they feel the required sorts of caring emotions.

Professional love does not have to be manufactured. It is skilled caring and the professional commitment to the welfare of the patient which is more important than searching one's inner depth for feelings (van Hooft 2006). Van Hooft goes further and criticises the way caring is taught:

> Nurse educators who seek to inculcate caring attitudes separately from such bodily comportment or professional commitment are still thinking in a dualistic manner.
>
> (van Hooft 2006, p. 105)

Nolan (2011) speaks of this attention, contained in presence as 'attending' and it can be part of any interaction and any clinical care if the nurse chooses to make it so. Presence and care are automatically demonstrated to a patient, in the body, the body language and 'comportment', of the nurse and midwife when they are committed to the patient's welfare, and acting professionally and caring skilfully and being authentic, because those beliefs will be embedded in their body. The patient will sense by their comportment, in other words, their demeanour, manner and conduct that they are cared about. This presence is spiritual because it is holistic, caring, loving and compassionate, the way spiritual beings are with each other, in order to be human, in the community of humanity.

Conclusion

Taylor's research led her to believe that there is a power in relationships that connects all of us to something spiritual. At the end of her study she had come to believe this:

> Rather like 'fairies in gumboots,' humans are interconnected, incarnate beings, with their feet weighted firmly to the ground. In living their daily routines they may have forgotten something of their spiritual heritage and their interconnectedness with all things but, thankfully, their forgetfulness is not entirely complete. The quality of their interpersonal relationships remind them now and then of the true beauty and power of their human existence.
>
> (Taylor 1994, p. 237)

Spiritual care through sharing, caring, attending, empathy and presence are practical ways to help you, in any context, to demonstrate compassion and by so doing affect the spirituality of others and enhance their spiritual well-being.

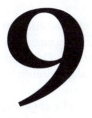

Talking about spirituality

Introduction

In this chapter the knotty issue of how it is possible to talk about spirituality and the place of spiritual assessment tools will be unpicked. The ways in which you can sustain the patient until their own resources can take over and how you can help to foster realistic hope will be explored. To do this you will need to be able to see and manage your own beliefs and values and how you can do this will be examined. Finally the role of the chaplain and the way it intersects with your role will end the chapter.

Getting to know someone's spiritual needs

While presence and compassionate care as Tanyi et al.'s study (2006) shows is recognised by patients as the most important part of spiritual care, sometimes patients in her study wanted to talk about their spiritual beliefs and some said they wanted the nurse to be able to initiate the discussion. So it is clear that in addition to caring and connecting as a way of giving spiritual care, spiritual care is also about being willing and able to listen when patients want to talk about issues related to their spirituality. Whether such discussions are nurse prompted will depend on what the nurse knows about the patient and their beliefs and background and the context of their illness and prognosis and whether the patient appears troubled. Any of these things could prompt you to explore with a patient their spiritual concerns. However, it should be borne in mind that some patients do not see this as the nurse's role and in Taylor and Mamier's (2005) study just over half her sample did not think it was the nurses' role. You are there in the capacity of a health-care worker and a patient's spiritual concerns are only your business if they somehow impact on the patients' health. There are depths of spiritual concern which only a specialist should be dealing with.

To talk about spirituality with someone you need to be engaged, interested and compassionate but patients don't generally expect you to display great knowledge of spirituality and religion. Nurses are travelling with patients and are not guides and it is perfectly acceptable to express ignorance but always alongside interest and a willingness to learn and to be with patients while they are learning how to deal with their confusion and fear when the things that made life meaningful are suddenly in disarray. To be authentic means admitting when you don't have the answer. The important thing is to be willing to stay with patients while they struggle to find the meaning they are seeking.

As has been explained earlier, just knowing that someone is ill, knowing their age, whether they have a mental health problem and knowing what they've said about their religion on admission will give you some clues as to what their quandaries about themselves and their life might be. Then noting their nationality, their language, if they live alone, if they have children and what their work is will also tell you something about them. Many encounters with patients are fleeting and the illness or injury they are confronting is unlikely to provoke spiritual concerns. Many other encounters are more long-lasting and repeated and do have implications for patients' spiritual well-being.

Nurses and midwives learn about patients' hopes, dreams, expectations, values, beliefs and how they live out their beliefs through getting to know them and relating to them as persons. Practitioners have to be able to create environments and relationships where patients feel free and confident to talk about personal issues when they want. To prompt a discussion about spirituality can feel daunting. Spirituality can be a difficult topic to talk about because it is so ambiguous and reactions to it can be very variable. Some people think about it a lot and some not at all. There is also a wide range of belief about the subject. It can help to start off with concrete and easily discussed questions and prompts whilst being open to when and if the patient wants to

move on to more personal beliefs. One patient in Tanyi et al.'s
study said:

> the easiest way is just to ask, and if they [patients] are open with
> it, that's fine, and if they are not, well that's another sign, too,
> that they, you know, that they have a different way of coping
> with things.
>
> (Tanyi et al. 2006, p. 535)

The most concrete aspect of spirituality is to do with religious
and spiritual beliefs, so that you could ask if someone thinks of
themselves as particularly religious or spiritual and this could lead
to a discussion about what practices they may have, which could
then lead to asking whether anything has changed recently in their
thinking. Another useful question is to ask what has helped them
most when they had crises and troubles in the past. Were any of
the practices they'd talked about helpful? Would they be helpful
now? If care is taken to always include the term 'spirituality' as
well as 'religion', it opens up the subject so that someone who
doesn't have a religious belief or whose faith has waned doesn't
feel excluded. As these issues are often seen as obscure, it can help
to use yourself as an example if you think someone doesn't understand what you mean. A nurse can explain what spirituality is by
explaining what it means to them.

Example

I'm a nurse on an oncology ward. When people come in and out for their
chemo, I often wonder who is looking after them in-between. You know,
when they're at home, not physically, but everything else that could be going
on. You can be so well between chemo treatments nowadays but you still
have cancer and people must worry so much about their future and there's
nobody around. Well nobody professional anyway and people often don't
want to talk to their family about that kind of thing. So I always try to get a bit
of time with them to see what they've got that's helping them really. I usually
just ask if they mind if we have a bit of a chat. I say that it's useful to have a
kind of personal store cupboard of resources to help them get through being
ill and ask if they think of themselves as being spiritual or religious in any
way. That starts things off and we talk about anything they want. Mostly I just
listen. It might be while I'm doing something else, like helping them wash,

if it seems right. They might talk about what they do, what they used to do, what they'd like to do. It might be anything from going to church to going for walks on the beach or talking to their husband. Often they talk about praying and whether it's worth it and they might talk about people they've lost touch with or argued with. I can't help with lots of things of course and they know that. I'm not a counsellor. So I keep them focused on what has helped in the past, will it help now and is there anything we can do to help them get back in touch with it. I can talk to them about life, the universe, God and every-thing ... to the extent that I have the same thoughts and feelings myself, after all I'm only human! – and if I have the time, but after that ... well, ... if they seem depressed or have a lot of questions or seem to have a deeper issue with their faith, I suggest they talk to the chaplain because they're special-ists and I'm not. It just seems to help to have someone acknowledge to them that illness does change how they think about lots of things and sometimes people have to find new ways of fitting things into place. They take it from there themselves.

Another participant in Tanyi et al.'s study said:

> Ask the person where they are [in their spiritual journey], and they'll go with it because everybody brings their own perspec-tive and judgment to a situation ... just help them try to get in touch with that entity that gets them through that minute.
>
> (Tanyi et al. 2006, p. 535)

Many of these kinds of prompts and questions have been formu-lated into tools which nurses can use. For instance the FICA tool focuses on four areas, 'Faith' and belief, the 'Importance' of this to the person, whether this means they are part of any partic-ular 'Community' and how they would like the practitioner to 'Address' any of these issues in their healthcare (Puchalski 2010). There are many such tools nurses could use as a guide to how the subject can be talked about to patients (see particularly Culliford and Eagger 2009, McSherry 2010, Puchalski 2010).

Some people suggest that patients should be formally assessed and the results documented; it may be that a formal assessment will alert the practitioner to issues that wouldn't have been picked up otherwise. Formal assessment is most often seen as part of the nursing process approach to spiritual care. However, against this is the fact that tools and questions might seem intrusive if used formally and could be a barrier to ordinary relationships.

Unfortunately formal spiritual assessment has come to be seen as almost definitive of spiritual care in recent years and to some authorities, if formal spiritual assessment is not taking place, it is assumed that spiritual care is also not taking place. As spiritual assessment is perceived as requiring time, education and competence beyond what most nurses think they have, there is a danger that nurses believe that they cannot or do not offer spiritual care because they cannot or do not feel able to conduct formal assessments. Whereas in fact there is plenty of evidence that spiritual care includes a much broader range of relational and caring activities than those activities that are likely to be implemented as a result of a spiritual assessment and in addition, much 'spiritual assessment' takes place during the course of informal caring (Taylor and Mamier 2005, Tanyi et al. 2006, McSherry and Jamieson 2011, Smyth and Allen 2011). An overemphasis on formal spiritual assessment has distracted nursing from more relational and embodied spiritual care and has been disempowering for nurses as it is seen as an insurmountable obstacle, so that its use, formally, for nurses is contentious (Johnson 2010). Nevertheless in selected circumstances, you may find more formal detailed and explicit assessment and recording of a person's spiritual history useful.

Sustaining: A concept borrowed from pastoral care

Christian pastoral care, the spiritual care that Christian chaplains give, has a history of 2000 years of helping people and there is scholarship and advice about how to do it going back almost as far. This is a classic definition of pastoral care:

> healing, sustaining, guiding, and reconciling of troubled persons whose troubles arise in the context of ultimate meanings and concerns.
>
> (Clebsch and Jaekle 1975, p. 4)

Whilst most of what Clebsch and Jaekle describe here would not be applicable to nurses, the function of 'sustaining' does helpfully describe a useful way of thinking when talking to and working with people who have suffered loss, whether through illness, bereavement, disability or, as Clebsch and Jaekle (1975) say, 'in any situation, where the sense dominates that all of life is running downhill' (p. 44). Sustaining, in this sense, means to support and hold someone up. It is not about solving the situation or having an answer but rather of keeping the person going until they can support themselves. They describe 'sustaining' (1975, p. 42) in four stages which should not be seen as necessarily linear.

Preservation – Helping someone to hold on to where they are and avoiding excessive retreat into despair. Illness, as has been seen earlier, involves loneliness and the feeling of being in a different land to those who are not ill, so that preservation could be seen metaphorically as grasping the person and just holding them where they are, including the person in the flow of life, so that they don't drift any further out to sea. This may just be in, as Clebsch and Jaekle say (1975, p. 45), 'a touch, a glance, a word a gesture'. Your aim is to reassure the person that they still belong, they are still anchored to their own life and identity, no matter what has happened or will happen. This might mean talking about the world outside the hospital and the illness, about their family and friends and about what is going on in the world. It also could be talking about the illness *with* the patient and not excluding them. Including them in decisions and reminding them that there are still decisions and choices they can make. Somehow, in preservation, the nurse is using their own resources and strength while the patients lie dormant. Just presence may be all that is possible at this point. Reminding the patient that they are not quite alone, they are still 'in' the world even though it doesn't feel like that now.

Consolation is, expressed by Clebsch and Jaekle as,

> to relieve one's sense of misery by bringing the sufferer into an understanding of his still belonging to the company of the hopeful living…(p. 45)…even while acknowledging that the damaging or robbing experience that initiated disconsolation remains irreparable.
>
> (1975, p. 47)

Morse et al. (1992) suggest that it is at this stage when comforting words can be used to encourage the person, which may only give some temporary relief – but they should not be disparaged because of that. They express the emotional engagement of the nurse, their care, and make visible their feelings and impulses to try to relieve suffering but with the full knowledge that it cannot be removed permanently. Morse et al. relate an incident of consolation from the experiences of Lear which took place in the waiting room of a Critical Care Unit after a husband and father had been admitted with a myocardial infarct:

> The nurse Bonnie came and went. Big Mama, so exquisitely attuned to countless women like me, whom she had consoled in the waiting room, that she seemed to be inside my head, to know exactly what images were trapped in there and how best to pet and soothe. Draping herself now about Judy and me, whispering news bulletins and cautionary notes: ' ... still holding his own ... we just don't know ... moment to moment ... ' I felt that I needed no cautions.
>
> (Lear 1980, cited by Morse et al. 1992)

Lear is duly cautioned about her loved husband's situation even through the soothing words.

Consolidation – This stage is about gathering resources and reviewing progress before moving forward. For the nurse this might be when the time is right to talk about what there still is left, what has been retained, when it's time to face the loss and meet it – time to place the loss within the perspective of the whole of life.

Redemption – To start to build a new life, to move forward. Time to talk about what is going to happen next, the future, how life is going to look now, how it will continue.

The crucial importance of hope

Hope is a thread that runs throughout the act of sustaining. Emphasis on speaking hopefully seems to have declined in nursing with the increased emphasis on honesty. Hope became associated with over-optimism and false hope. However, it is central to spiritual well-being (Clark et al. 1991, Tanyi 2002) and to being able to find meaning in illness (Post-White et al. 1996), so that nurses and midwives have to find ways to be hopeful whilst not being deceitful or raising expectations unrealistically. Hope is about desiring and envisioning a positive future or a positive outcome, which does not have to mean envisioning cure. A positive future could mean hoping that the new analgesia will work better than the last, or hope that sleeplessness will disappear. Hope may be in getting back to work, planning a holiday; having a good life despite what has happened. Or it may be hope for a painless and calm death. Hope may also rest in what will happen after your death, in the hope that your children will have happy and successful lives or that a partner will recover quickly and find new happiness. Hope may be that the memories you leave behind will be good ones and that what you achieved in your lifetime will be long-lasting. Any of these things may be worked towards and can give a sense of hope and improvement to come as well as a sense of success and achievement. Being able to envisage that the people you leave behind have been enriched because of your life, or that your achievements in your career have left a positive effect can add richness to your own life and make life seem more meaningful. Research with patients and carers suggest that warm, caring relationships help to foster hope in people (Clark et al. 1991) as does bringing time horizons closer so that hope is in the next hour or day rather than the distant future. To be given something humorous or distracting to think about or to envisage or experience a hopeful image like a sunset, or listening to inspiring music also fosters hope and practitioners can encourage patients to make use of these kinds of things (Herth 1993).

For many people their hope may be in the belief that death is not the complete end, and even those who do not profess to a formal religion may have this underlying belief or feeling. Whatever the nurse may feel, such hope should always be fostered and allowed to flourish as the outcome of this kind of hope can never be known. Hope has to be meaningful and futile and fervent hope of recovery can be an obstacle to spiritual well-being as it can lead to disappointment and despair. Hope which is clearly known to be unrealistic may prevent development of hope in things that can be achieved. When someone can be helped to begin to adjust their hopes onto more realistic aims it is usually because they have managed to reach some readjustment of expectations and accepted the changed meaning of their life (Watson et al. 2009). However, each person is on their own journey at their own pace and nurses, while encouraging more meaningful hope, cannot force someone to move more quickly than they are ready to.

Managing your own spirituality and talking about yourself

In developing relationships with patients that enables care to be spiritual, nurses need to be authentic and to present themselves to a patient as a whole person as Buber describes. As with any aspect of life, we take with us into any relationship, our knowledge and understanding about life and the experiences we have had. The experiences of life which have affected a nurse's spiritual outlook can be helpful to them in understanding what patients may be going through, so anything which helps you to bring these to mind can be helpful to developing empathy with patients. Knowledge about spirituality is useful to be able to understand what patients may be experiencing and knowledge about your own values and beliefs is useful to be able to see others in perspective and in order to make contrasts and understand differences. But this kind of knowledge and understanding can come in many different ways; not just by going on a course or a study day.

Example

I really try to listen to patients and give them my whole attention when I'm looking after them but then I try to do that when I'm with friends too come to think about it. Patients sometimes have some quite deep questions they want to talk about when they're ill and all you can do is just make it clear that you'd like to listen if they want to talk and then just shut up and listen. I don't remember anyone ever telling me that. I've picked up a lot through just nursing people and watching how other people do it. I remember seeing how one ward sister calmed down this really angry old man by just focusing on him and talking really quietly then just listening to him. It turned out he was angry because he was so upset about being ill and thought it meant the end of his independence, he blamed God for letting him get old, said he couldn't see the point. I've also picked up a lot by being married. When my husband's upset or angry, he just wants me to listen to him. He hates it when I interrupt him to tell him what's what. 'You have to stop thinking that you have to have all the answers', he said to me once. He's just like a lot of patients really. We all want the same things in the end don't we. I used to meditate and read a bit about spiritual techniques, I think that helped because I did learn a lot about being 'in the moment'. I don't do it now . . . but maybe I'll get back into it again. You do kind of think sometimes that you have to have a way to deal with all the sadness you see in this job.

Nurses and patients are all, in effect, journeying together and patients are more trusting of nurses who admit that they don't have all the answers and have the confidence to behave with ordinariness.

Being human and whole means that you take all your own beliefs and values into each encounter with you. If you are being authentic you will always be acting out of your values whether you are aware of it or not and it is not possible or desirable for anyone to have to 'divide themselves off from their faith' when they go to work (Pollard 2009). As a patient in Tanyi et al.'s study said about nurses, 'I feel that when they get involved, their spirituality shows through and you just kind of know and you can see it' (2006, p. 535).

What this suggests is that the practitioner's spirituality is part of their being, and it is interpreted by patients as being as much about what you do and who you are as what you believe and what you say. Your own spiritual beliefs are less important than whether you act out of compassion and care for others. Compassion is more important than striving to rigidly follow the rules and principles that come from your beliefs (Clarke 2011). Most people have strong beliefs about life and this may include religious belief therefore it is important to understand and respect the differences between people. It might be very hard for an atheist to understand why someone might choose a course of action based on a religious belief but they have to accept it when it is part of their professional role to do so. If you are finding it difficult to support someone in making a decision that clashes with your own beliefs, you need to talk about it to someone like your manager or the chaplain or a trusted friend and, if necessary, ask to be removed from the situation. However, it is often at times of disagreement when patients and nurses have the most opportunities to learn something which helps everyone on their own path. You could sit quietly with a patient and tell them that you're finding it difficult to understand why they are making a particular decision because you don't believe the same things as them. Being open to others with different beliefs shows how much you care about them; asking them to help you to understand why they believe what they do can help the patient to clarify their decision for themselves and show them that you are genuinely respectful and interested. Having a belief system of your own can help you understand difference and to appreciate other people's beliefs, but if patients start to perceive it as a barrier to relationship and communication then you need to discuss it with someone to find a way of working and believing, which patients will be able to accept.

The focus of care is the patient and your aim will be to allow each person to have the confidence and freedom to talk about their own spiritual beliefs and feelings. However, sometimes a patient will ask you about yours or the issue will come up in conversation and then it's okay to answer briefly and honestly. Patients usually appreciate honesty and in most studies about care, patients say that it's important to them in building relationships that nurses disclose something about themselves. Patients sometimes feel that it is reassuring to know that you have beliefs even if they don't hold those beliefs themselves as it makes you look like a whole, real human being. However, you have to always be aware that patients may be feeling insecure and searching for something to believe in at times of stress, and it would be wrong to take advantage of the relationship to try to persuade patients that your beliefs are right. This is called proselytising, and it is a misuse of your role.

It is part of some religions to pray for people; people you know or don't know and whole countries and groups. Parish priests pray for all the people in their parish every day whether they are of the same religion or not and in churches the whole country is prayed for. Prayer for some people is a very big part of Christian worship so it would not be surprising if Christian nurses prayed for all their patients each day and they may even pray for particular people. If you do this you have to remember that you must adhere to confidentiality guidelines and not mention publicly any names or other details about a person in your care. If you're considering whether to tell a person that you are praying for them or to ask a patient if they would like to be prayed for, you have to use your judgement based on your knowledge of the patient and your relationship with them to decide whether it would help them to know or whether it would be irrelevant or even a hindrance to your relationship with them. Some people, especially if they have the same belief system would be very heartened to know they are being prayed for. For others, it might cause confusion, stress or even anger. When you know a patient very well and understand their beliefs and know that they pray too, you may want to suggest praying together, but you would have to know a patient very well before you did this and be confident as to how the suggestion would be received. Praying *with* patients would usually only happen if it is suggested by the patient themselves (Narayanasamy and Narayanasamy 2008). If a patient asks you to pray with them and you don't want to you could cause hurt or embarrassment by simply refusing. To be given such a request is a privilege and it shows the patient has trust in you. An alternative to a refusal is to explain how you feel but ask to stay with the patient while *they* pray. To a person who is used to prayer, the solidarity of having another person with them who they feel close to can be supportive, but this doesn't mean you have to share the same beliefs.

When you confront a dilemma with a patient you can also be affected and feel that you have grown spiritually or you may feel confronted with a question that you haven't had to consider before. This can be uncomfortable. When you open yourself to other people you may experience very profound moments or some uncomfortable confusing challenges. It is usually in those moments that the most intense emotional connections can occur. It is very important that if you feel disturbed or uncomfortable you seek out someone to talk about it. A good person may be a chaplain; remember that the chaplain's role is to support staff as well as patients, and the role of the chaplain will be spoken of later in this chapter. This doesn't mean that anything is wrong, on the contrary, but even positive moments can be uncomfortable and confusing.

Conventional wisdom dictates that nurses who commit themselves or connect too deeply with patients risk 'burnout'. But, in a study involving interviews with 35 intensive care nurses, Leppanen-Montgomery (1991) found that those who experienced a sense of connection to a force greater than themselves in the relationship were able to achieve closeness and commitment without risk of burnout. Instead they experienced fulfilment and growth. The union they achieved with patients was, they said, 'beyond the level of self, at the level of spirit' (p. 95) and it was not felt as over personalised and excessive. A crucial characteristic of nurses who achieved relationships of what she called 'spiritual transcendence' was that their aim was simply to connect with patients and they didn't have any other agenda or expectation. The nurses in the study, who had negative experiences of their job, especially dealing with death, were those who did not achieve any sense of transcendence and these nurses tended to be those with no spiritual resources. They experienced only anguish and ultimately chose to distance themselves from their work in order to cope. The implications of this are that it is not having spiritual awareness that is important but rather having spiritual resources which can fortify and sustain you so that you can take the risk of real relationships with patients. Just as with patients this kind of resource may take the form of relationships with family and friends; a place to let off steam and feel confirmed. It could be confirming and connecting activities like exercise and pursuing hobbies and interests. It could be having a philosophical or spiritual framework that enables you to deal with being confronted with your own mortality as well as the threat of pain and disability that you see in patients (Leppanen-Montgomery 1991). This is one area that employers and universities should focus on if nurses and midwives are to be enabled to develop spiritual care.

Thinking time

Spend a few minutes on your own now thinking about what your beliefs about the world are. Do you believe in any kind of spiritual power? How does this affect the way you live? What resources or help do you have which will help you in a crisis or an illness?

The role of the chaplain

One of the ways in which nurses and midwives can help people towards wholeness and finding meanings in their illness is by referral to the chaplain. The chaplaincy service in the NHS has changed considerably in recent years from having only a Christian and religious function to become a spiritual care service available to everyone, regardless of their beliefs. In addition chaplains are specialists in religion in general and their own religion in particular. Chaplains are now expected to take the lead in NHS Trusts in promoting spiritual care in which all people regardless of their spiritual beliefs or faith have the right to have those beliefs respected. Chaplains aim to help people to find wholeness and interconnection with an emphasis on the fullness and totality of the person and as such their aims are the same as other health practitioners as regards spirituality (Newitt 2010). However, they have a different role and different skills to nurses and midwives. Chaplains interact with patients predominantly outside their clinical management, and so they are sometimes more able to stand outside the system and alongside the patient as an advocate. Their specialist skills in pastoral care of which there is a very long tradition enables them to talk more easily about spirituality and as it is their main role, they are likely to have more time to focus on talking and listening. Whereas nurses and midwives might have less time to talk, but they are present with patients for longer periods and when they are at their most vulnerable and they have the opportunity for physical care which chaplains don't have. You should therefore be prepared to refer patients to chaplains, not only because they have specific religious needs but when they have spiritual needs which require more prolonged conversation and more experienced and specialist skills than you yourself are able to give. Chaplains are also specialists in liturgy and are able to help people use rituals to mark transitions and events in their life. Just because someone doesn't declare themselves to be part of a recognised religion doesn't mean they don't have religious beliefs. As has been explained, religious belief these days is much more fluid than it once was and Chaplains are skilled in helping people to identify, clarify and express their beliefs without asserting any pressure to choose any particular religion or institution. They can work creatively with people to write prayers and liturgy when the traditional means available in the orthodox religions don't seem to fit their needs. There are often chaplains available from a variety of different religions. The needs that people have are very diverse, especially in today's society where there are many people who find that they need some means of thanking, worshipping, asking forgiveness of, raging against or imploring a deity when they don't believe in or belong to a formal religion. For instance Newitt (2010, p. 172) describes how he increasingly finds he needs a form of prayer to help people in 'making peace with a God you are not sure exists'. Grace Davie who researches religion in Britain relates the experience of a hospital chaplain in Liverpool who cared for women patients in two different hospitals. One group was older, their problems were often with cancer, and they seemed to have more ability to express their spiritual beliefs and emotions, be they joy or anger because they remembered their early church experiences and some of the language of prayer and ritual. The younger group, who were giving birth or dealing with miscarriage or infertility, born since the 1960s, did not know how to communicate with the chaplain, and had no spiritual or religious language to recall when they needed it, to help them express their spiritual longings and feelings to and about God. The chaplain had to help them to find new forms of communicating with what they perceived as a God (Davie 1994). Nevertheless both groups were equally pleased to see the chaplain, and as Davie said, 'Indeed in both hospitals there were repeated expressions of gratitude that there was someone in the institution whose business it was to affirm joy, to assuage grief and to comfort in times of tribulation' (Davie 1994, p. 123).

Conclusion

Talk should not be the whole of spiritual care but it is a crucial part of it for many patients. It is in talking about spirituality and listening to another person tell you about their own spiritual beliefs, cares and worries that you perhaps need to particularly remember about being ordinary; remember that there is not such a big difference between you and them and that your own experiences can help you in understanding others. You can't make problems go away but you can give the gift of yourself in helping to hold up another person with consoling words, encouragement and hope until they are strong enough for their own resources to take over.

Part IV
Making Physical Care Spiritual

10 Comfort and care of the body

Introduction

People usually live with their body in the background of their lives not in the foreground. They are not conscious of their bodies as they live their lives day by day; bodies are silent and largely forgotten most of the time, until they choose to force themselves on our awareness (van Manen 1998). Events such as illness or disability bring the body into consciousness, into the foreground of our life. When something goes wrong with the body it also becomes the concern of others as well as yourself and the body that you identify as your 'self' becomes an object to other people and, to some extent, an object that is separated from you.

> It is indeed a painful experience when, as a patient, one feels as if the sick body has become a thing at the disposal of the medical workers rather than a thing which is meaningfully integrated in one's own life projects.
>
> (van Manen 1998, p. 10)

Sometimes it's necessary to cultivate this point of view when, for instance, you are in intractable pain. However, having your body as an object which other people are observing, measuring and discussing can make you feel fragmented and when you feel fragmented it's as if your body and soul are disconnected from each other, as if you are literally in pieces, the self in conflict with the body (Cassell 2004). Medicine tends to deal with the body as an object but caring can protect the whole person from being treated as an object. A person who is not able to be in control of their own surroundings and even their own body suffers a loss in their integrity which is often expressed as a loss of dignity

(Gadow 1985), whereas a person who is in control, who is treated as a whole person and not as an object, has dignity. This chapter and the ones that follow will focus on what it means to have a body that we have lost control over, that is fragmented and sick. First there will be an analysis from what patients say their body feels like when it is sick. This will be followed by a glance back into history to explore how nurses have given physical care and provided comfort in the past with a comparison to how physical care rates in our priorities now. Then there will be an exploration of how comfort can be given and what patients say it makes them feel like. Lastly a section is devoted to old people because old people face particular challenges in exposing their body to the world and young people face particular challenges in nursing them.

The sick body

Nurses frequently say they are going to make someone 'comfortable' to refer to different things from moving someone to giving them analgesia. In the previous chapter, the breadth of the term 'comfort' was explored as well as how the root of the word means 'to strengthen', suggesting that the idea of comfort could have far-reaching meaning for the spiritual aspects of care which aims to strengthen the person's spirit to be able to manage their present circumstances. Morse et al. (1995) tried to discover what this concept actually meant to patients and found that although comfort was hard for people to describe, it was recognised when it was suddenly there in contrast to its opposite, discomfort. Comfort is something that most of the time people are not conscious of and it seems like feeling integrated, everything just feels all right (Morse et al. 1995). Almost all experiences of illness or injury are about feeling not only that bodies are broken, but also that *how you feel about* your body is also broken. People feel let down by their body and this contributes to feelings of disintegration which is not only about the body 'falling apart' but of body and self dis-integrating, becoming separated. To long to be well is to long to be whole again.

From in-depth, unstructured interviews with 36 people who were dealing with serious illnesses and traumatic injuries, Morse et al. (1995) built up a picture of how a sick person's relationship with their body changes and how feelings of separation between body and self happens. It is as if people take on a series of different bodies which take the place of the one they used to know: the *dis-eased body, the disobedient body, deceiving body, the vulnerable body, the violated body, the enduring body, the resigned body* and the *betraying body.*

The *dis-eased* body begins to appear as symptoms like tiredness, stiffness, pain and an array of other sensations start to irritate and interfere with what you want to do. The body starts to look like a burden or an obstacle sitting in front of us, in our way. Every new sensation causes worry, it may be innocent or sinister. The body starts to demand attention and puts itself centre stage, you can no longer forget your body and increasingly you just don't feel like yourself (Morse et al. 1995). Öhman et al. (2003) also studied the experiences of chronically ill patients using narrative interviews with ten people. They spoke of how the body starts to become an obstacle, filled with pain, preventing independence and robbing autonomy. One participant said, 'you become slight and insignificant' (Öhman et al. 2003, p. 533).

The *disobedient* body describes the realisation that your body can't be commanded any longer and it seems less and less under your control. No matter how much willpower you exert, you can be suddenly struck by diarrhoea, paralysis, tiredness and incontinence at the most inconvenient and embarrassing times, so that your body seems not to belong to you anymore. It seems completely separate to your mind.

The *deceiving* body looks and feels just the same but under the surface insidious changes are taking place. So when the disease is finally revealed, you feel angry that your body has let you down. You had trusted it and all the time it was secretly deceiving you.

The *vulnerable* body is filled with fear about the treatments and assaults that may come soon – from surgery to the hurdles of the first bath after a mastectomy or the first sight of a wound. You can start to feel at the mercy of the doctors, nurses and therapists who surround you. Although you know that they are there to help, the people around you are actually causing you more pain and indignity which adds to the feelings of fear and danger. One woman in Morse et al.'s study said:

They would come in and set all their trays up (for burn debridement) and the minute you hear those metal trays (you) start shaking, your stomach gets all in knots and you're scared because you know the pain that's going to be coming.

(Morse et al. 1995, p. 17)

The patients in Öhman et al.'s (2003) study also talked about treatments that added to suffering and made them feel worse. This can leave patients feeling defenceless and the drive to protect the body from such assaults can lead to treatment being refused.

The *violated* body expresses how patients feel exposed and embarrassed by the intrusions into their privacy that they are forced to experience. They feel they have lost their dignity and the respect of those around them. Morse et al. (1995) describe how the way practitioners talk aloud about your symptoms and ask personal questions as routine 'Have you had your bowels open today', for instance, can feel as though your privacy is being invaded. However, despite the embarrassment and outrage, patients still consent to procedures and examinations because they know it is necessary if they are to get well. They also know that sometimes it helps to see their own body as an object when that is the only way to detach themselves from pain and indignity when a particularly painful or embarrassing procedure is taking place such as with this interviewee.

In the hospital it's like you have no rights, you have no say, you don't even have power over your own body. I had a hard time … when five doctors come in at the same time … and they talk(ed) about you like you're a piece of meat. And they want to see, of course, where you are burned and how your scars are healing. Well, you have to flip up your gown so everybody can see, and it's just an awful feeling. You lose your modesty as well as – your dignity? And after a while of that you just don't care, you start thinking of yourself as a piece of meat, that's all.

(Morse et al. 1995, p. 17)

However, sometimes the only way for someone to endure an embarrassing or painful situation is for them to try to objectify their body, to see it as separate from themselves. In those moments the nurse can use their communication skills in 'their voices, eyes and hands' to help people to give up a bit of themselves and still maintain their dignity (Morse et al. 1995, p. 192).

The *enduring* body has given in to the pain and discomfort and reluctantly accepts it as a fact of present life. Just being able to endure their lives is the only option left. Endurance has the element of acceptance but not a willing acceptance.

The *betraying* body is the body that shows the signs of stress and depression when the patient is working hard to put on a positive face and to look as though they're coping. The tension shows in muscle tightness, indigestion, insomnia. While the body has seemed to be out of the control of the mind up to this point, it now seems as though it was being controlled by your mind after all but at a much deeper level than the conscious will. The body betrays your state of mind when you would rather your state of mind was hidden (Morse et al. 1995).

The *resigned* body shows itself when a change becomes permanent; the body is permanently changed so that it no longer fits the image you have of it, it seems to be in conflict with one's identity. It has been forced to give in to the inevitable and no matter what the self wills, the body will not comply. There is a sense of permanent loss; there will be no recovery of that particular function, this particular thing will not change (Morse et al. 1995).

What the nurse is trying to achieve in their care of people with sick and dis–integrated bodies is what van Manen calls 'meaningful, worthwhile, and liveable relations between the physical body and the lived body, between the embodied being and the world' (van Manen 1998, p. 17). What the next section shows is that nurses may have had more tools to do this work in the past than they do now.

A short history of physical comfort in nursing

When Carole Estabrooks (1987) compared nursing literature from the first 20 years of the 20th century with nursing literature from the period 1970–1985 to see how touching the body was dealt with, she found some interesting differences. Whereas the idea of carrying out procedures was just as common in both sets of data, the idea of doing something *for* the patient's comfort was not. Estabrooks found that nurses in the early 20th century seemed to engage in much more physical and personal care and used touch and bathing in much more therapeutic ways than present-day nurses seem to do. Hydrotherapy was fashionable in the early 20th century and was considered an effective treatment for so many ailments that nurses learnt how to offer many different types of bath. However, they were not only carrying out prescribed treatments by doctors; they recognised the therapeutic use of bathing in itself as a nursing activity and not only to clean the skin and reduce fever. Estabrooks quotes from Crawford from 1910:

> I have concluded that baths are given, first, for cleanliness or to remove dirt and dead epithelium; second, as an antipyretic or to reduce fever; third, to stimulate the function of the skin by reaction , increase the activity of the respiratory and circulatory organs; fourth, as a sedative.
>
> (Crawford 1910, p. 314)

Nurses today would probably only see the bath as useful for the first reason, for hygiene. They are more likely to give paracetamol or aspirin to reduce a pyrexia; they would probably never see a bath as a way to help the circulatory or respiratory systems (and whether it would is debatable) and would seldom use it as a sedative. In their own homes, most people if they were hot might take a cool bath, but nurses today would probably balk at the idea of helping a patient into a bath when they have a high temperature and helping them into water that was less than warm would surely infringe some health and safety rule. But bathing is a way to calm down and relax; again, it's what many would do in their own homes. But how often would a nurse in a hospital recommend it for that reason? They are more likely to ask a doctor to prescribe a sedative. In fact the term 'sedation' has become synonymous with taking medication. You could construe from this that nurses in an earlier era whilst having less autonomy in some ways perhaps had more autonomy with regard to their own practice and more therapeutic tools within their own control than nurses do currently. The idea that bathing could be a useful therapeutic tool for reasons other than cleanliness seems to be lost. For instance, in most textbook procedures these days hygiene is the only rationale suggested for bathing (Woods 2011). It seems that when nurses bathed patients in 1903 there was much more recognised as happening, than in 2012. Gordon in 1903 said,

let the patient regard the process with pleasure.... Endeavour
to be an artist in sponging.... Know why you sponge.... Let
your touch be gentle, firm, and soothing.

(Gordon 1903, p. 595).

Estabrooks (1987) talks of how in this early literature gentleness was emphasised in any caring activity, whether it be bathing
or turning and moving a patient. Massage was much used and
encouraged but with the proviso, as today, that some massage
should be left to a trained masseur. The artistry of nursing
was much more in evidence in this era and it was unashamedly
celebrated in this literature.

In comparing the way touch was spoken of or implied in
the historical literature Estabrooks (1987) found that there were
two types of touch used which she calls procedural and comfort
touch. Procedural touch means touch which occurs during other
activities and comfort touch means solely to provide comfort.
Today procedural touch is more likely to be called instrumental
or task touch, whilst touch which is not related to procedures
is called affective, expressive and non-procedural. This might be
thought to relate to the 'comfort' touch found in the historical literature. However, Estabrooks notes a profound difference
that in the historical literature, comfort touch was performed
with the intent to provide comfort, while the 'affective, expressive
and non-procedural touch' found in modern nursing is generally
something which is not deliberately performed for comfort, but
is incidental and peripheral to the main procedure and not necessary for accomplishing the task. An examination of a range of
British clinical procedure textbooks published in 2011 shows that
this difference still exists. In today's clinical procedure textbooks,
touch and the possibility of it having a positive effect in itself is
rarely mentioned (for instance, see Woods 2011, procedure for
a bed bath). Ideas such as those expressed by Gordon above in
1903 seem to be absent from the instructions we give today to
student nurses. Touch as a way of transmitting care is forgotten,
as is the idea that bathing can be any more than a mechanical
procedure for removing debris from the skin. The dominant discourse of 'the procedure' is scientific medicalism, which is about
efficient routes to medical outcomes rather than interpersonal relationships. In this paradigm, 'Good caring is routine, ritualized
tasks practiced on patients passive bodies' (Grant et al. 2005,

p. 502). Grant found that student nurses faced dilemmas when they attempted to construct care from different discourses which required empathy, warmth, common sense and humanism as these just didn't fit with the routines of care. Comfort as an aim in itself has disappeared from our horizon and clinical procedures, such as bathing, seem to have become dominated by mechanistic and scientific aims.

It may be that this lack of focus on ordinary physical comfort has contributed to the neglect of ordinary acts of physical care that patients complain of. It seems to have slipped down the list of priorities. As Estabrooks (1987) concluded, in modern nursing, the idea of carrying out a task with the sole aim of providing 'comfort' seems to have been forgotten (Estabrooks 1987). For instance, today in the Royal Marsden Hospital Manual of Clinical Nursing Procedures (Dougherty and Lister 2011), perhaps the most referred to manual for clinical care, the section on 'Patient Comfort' of some 114 pages consists of guidelines on a variety of 'procedures' from bed bath and various eye care procedures through to epidural catheter maintenance, and the application of compression garments; with no mention of comfort for the sake of comfort. It is as if we have come to believe that if we divided the person into their physiological parts and applied the correct hygiene and body maintenance procedure to the right part that 'comfort' would, in the terminology of nursing, be 'covered'. However, what patients call comfort does not appear to be written in any of these procedures; although when it exists, it exists in them all, and all the time, outside them all.

Thinking time

Remember the talk in the previous chapters about attention and presence and care? If you brought that knowledge into what you do when you give a bed bath, what would it be like?

Imagine for a few moments what it would be like for the patient.

Now imagine what it would be like for you.

'Let me make you comfortable'

Comfort is a thread that is embroidered into all the relationships that nurses and midwives have and woven into all the tasks of physical care. Bottorff found this when she asked patients about what it is like to be comforted by a nurse:

> Sandy [the nurse midwife] was wonderful. I remember her touching my legs after the baby was born and after the placenta was delivered...She touched my legs and rubbed my feet a little bit...Nobody ever did that to me... since I was really little and my mother rubbed my feet for me.
>
> (Patricia) (Bottorff 1991, p. 246)

It is particularly in providing physical comfort which is not necessary to the task which seems to evoke the strongest feelings of connection, transcendence and well-being when you know you are being cared for beyond the requirements of the clinical procedure. Like Ruth describes here when an injection becomes much more than a way to give a drug,

> I laid in my bed and she'd talk to me and she sat on the bed with me and then she did the needle. But before she did the needle she would rub the area and warm it up and she talked about my skin to me. It was just a whole different experience. And then she said, 'I imagine that was painful for you. I think you deserve a back rub for that.' So she gave me a wonderful back rub. It was just so nurturing.
>
> (Ruth) (Bottorff 1991, p. 242)

As well as the consequences for patients in the neglect of comfort, there are also consequences for nurses. By not valuing and celebrating the significance of touch and physical care to provide comfort, nurses are denying themselves an important tool for therapeutic nursing which is part of the uniqueness of nursing. Nurses who use touch as an essential aspect of physical care and not just incidental to it could rediscover a new tool in therapeutic nursing which not only benefits patients but which is empowering for nurses. Aside from the fact that nurses have such an array of opportunities to use physical care and touching to develop relationships which are spiritually nurturing that are not open to other professionals, they can also use the more deliberate and skilled ways of touch such as massage in their daily work (Tutton 1998). When providing comfort moves from the incidental to the deliberate, patients become aware that nurses are focused on them and 'going the extra mile' (Fosbinder 1994) and this is often achieved by the deliberate use of touch. Edvardsson et al. (2003) taught a group of nurses specific touching and massage skills to use with elderly people and then asked the nurses how it had affected their role. They all reported changes to their feelings about being a nurse. They suddenly felt like:

> a valuable person and professional... who is no longer power-less in the face of older patients haunted and disrupted bodies, but one who, by means of touch, has gained power to ease this suffering.
>
> (Edvardsson 2003, p. 606)

These nurses felt that the deliberate use of touch had deepened their relationships with patients and helped them to see the patient more as a person; they felt they had matured as professionals. In giving touch, concepts of body and self, doing and being and I and You, are brought together into one act (Edvardsson 2003).

In a study about spiritual care when patients were asked what specific events contributed to their sense of well-being and hope, many patients cited acts of physical care. One patient said, 'she massaged my back and rubbed my legs with lotion. Her touch was soothing, rhythmical, and gentle. I felt strength coming from the nurse' (Clark et al. 1991).

The old body

The young often seem to believe that the older person is not aware of the negative views generally held in society about the older person's body. The older people in Twigg's (2000) study however seemed well aware of it and their shame was acute. One patient felt 'dreadful' at having to expect a young pretty nurse to bathe them (Twigg 2000, p. 60). Whitaker (2010) found that with age, aware-ness of the body comes more to the fore in the minds of older people whereas to the rest of society ageing bodies are objects of rejection and denial. Even the oldest old say that they are acutely aware of the look and feel of their own body and their sense of themselves is still very much influenced by the way their body is managed and touched by other people (Whitaker 2010). The increasing needs and demands of the older body and its inexorable and visible progress towards death mean that it becomes central to how older people experience their being in the world. So that as they progressively hand over more of their body to others for care, how that care is performed has a crucial part to play in the spiritual life of older adults because sensitive touch and care restores dignity and personhood. When Whitaker conversed with and observed residents of a nursing home from the age of 71–101 over a period of seven months to explore how they were experiencing life generally, she found that the dominating topic of their lives was their body, how it is declining and how death is nearer (Whitaker 2010). They were living with varying levels of pain and dependence yet most perceived themselves as aiming to get well. Their shame and embarrassment at incontinence and dependence was as acute as any young person's might be. They wanted clean teeth and nails and fresh attractive clothes and hair as much as any younger person. Yet they were aware of how dependent they were on others for these things and could remember, if nothing else, a time of attraction and stamina. One woman of 99 says, 'I can't believe it's true, how old I am, and wrinkly, and dirty . . . no, not dirty but . . . Do you think I'm wrinkly?' (Whitaker 2010, p. 100). Another says, 'This . . . look here!' [she lifts her arm and slaps the sagging skin of her upper arm] 'This was once me; those are the remains of my past self' (p. 100). These elderly people identified themselves with their body but at the same time they knew that a body that was ageing and sick was a threat to their sense of themselves and so they tried to distance themselves from what their body meant. Their bodies had become to some extent appropriated by other agencies, 'owned by the staff' of the nursing home (Whitaker 2010, p. 102). It is as if beyond a certain age the body somehow became public property. Nurses will often have heard the resigned patient who declares, 'You can do with me what you like, I'm past caring'.

Older people are as concerned with their identity as anyone else and have, if anything, a greater need to experience life to the full, to become full people, in the limited time they have left. Their world may perhaps have dwindled down to the space they themselves inhabit, in a society which increasingly wishes to deny their very existence. Sadly older people living alone or in nursing homes may never feel the touch of another person unless it is instrumental yet their need to be touched may be greater than ever because most other sensual experiences have faded. To Whitaker (2010, p. 102), the residents she got to know, needed to have their bodies confirmed and touched 'beyond the instrumental and task-oriented "bed and body" work', just as much or more than anyone else.

Conclusion

In holistic spiritual care which aims to help patients to integrate, connect and feel whole, care of the body cannot be ignored. Understanding the importance of the body to spiritual care and reclaiming comfort and nursing ways to provide comfort will empower nurses and midwives as well as providing a truly spiritual style of personal care. The next chapter will explore in more detail the centre of spiritual, physical care, the subject of touch.

11 Touch and touching

Introduction

The philosopher David Levin, building on the ideas of Merlau Ponty about the body, explains that the meaning of who we are, our essential nature is written in the body. He suggests that when appropriate care is used in the handling of the body, when it is related to as though it is a whole person, that the true nature of that whole person is allowed to become manifest. He compares this with the 'grasping' touch of our technological age which is powerful but which cannot reach the true nature of things. Illness forces people to go through the treadmill of exposure, examination, diagnosis and treatment and interminable tests. These attacks make us feel bruised and psychologically battered, before we are healed. The opposite of this is the 'careful touch'.

> The careful touch, which is open to feeling what it touches and uses, gets in touch with a thing's essential nature more deeply and closely than the hand which wilfully grasps and clings, moved by strong desires (i.e. by attractions and aversions), or than the hand which is indifferent to the beauty of the thing in the wholeness of its truth.
>
> (Levin 1985, p. 128)

The strong desires Levin talks of could be the pressure to get the patient to do what *we* want. In this chapter, how to use this 'care full' touch so as to get 'in touch' with the real person beneath your hands will be explored and related to how a person feels about themselves. The types of touch and the meaning of touch and the array of personal preferences and how these are noted and included by picking up cues and clues will then be explored. Next, the role that touch can play in mental health nursing will be discussed.

Touching the body and touching the person

Being conscious and aware of the person being touched are essential to this act of getting in touch with the true nature of the person under our touch and in our care. This is also associated with a readiness to put aside our own desires and their 'attractions and aversions'. It includes a willingness to feel and appreciate the difference and individuality of each person and to try to see the beauty of them as we hold them in our hands. Levin reminds us that by handling anything 'tactfully' we leave it 'in-tact' and whole (1985, p. 129).

Touch seems to have the power to affect how a person feels about themselves. Gadow explains how practitioners can restore a person to being a subject and help them to feel like a whole person again, just by how they touch the very surface of someone's body. A surface touch can have a deep effect such that it is like a 'calling forth of the self' (Gadow 1985, p. 40), literally coaxing someone back to themselves. Gadow uses a phrase from a Richard Wilbur poem to describe how touch can expose 'the soul unshelled' (1985, p. 40). She goes on to say,

> Among all forms of human interaction, touch is the reminder that objectivity is not even skin deep. In touch, subjectivity exists at the surface of the body, and health professionals understand this perfectly.
>
> (Gadow 1985, p. 40)

When someone is physically touched they immediately respond, subjectively, as a whole person and in a more powerful way than if they hear or see. As Gadow says, nurses who use touch know that touching someone can bring them back to a sense of themselves. Touch is more personal and more intrusive than other sensations therefore you are more vulnerable when you are touched. The effect of touch on a person is so profound that practitioners are well aware that they have to take into account a variety of cultural and personal rules about touch which don't exist for hearing or seeing. There are rules and rituals in all cultures about who can and who cannot be touched, when and in what way. Even getting close to touching is considered hazardous so that personal space is considered crucial; we have all had the experience of stepping back when we felt someone was too close.

Types of touch

The distinction between necessary and non-necessary touch which has been made since 1970s. tends to ignore the fact that during necessary, procedural touch, emotions may also be expressed. While a nurse is putting the blood pressure cuff on a patient's arm, they can touch a patient, carefully or carelessly, gently or roughly, with attention or distractedly and all these things will be communicated to the patient. Practitioners who come into touching contact with patients may only touch them instrumentally but that instrumental touch is also expressive and one action can include various types of touch.

Van Manen (1999, p. 12) makes a similar distinction between pathic and gnostic touch. While gnostic touch is the touch of diagnosis, palpation and probing, pathic touch is 'supportive, caring, comforting, healing and therapeutic'. Pathic touch exploits the propensity for touch to enable someone to feel their own body and also removes the distance between the touched and the toucher, 'one is invited to inhabit one's own body' (p. 12).

The distinction between types of touch would become even more blurred if nurses were to return to using physical care therapeutically so that they consciously choose to use a bed bath, a foot soak, or a foot or hand massage, just to provide comfort as nurses in 1910 were apparently doing.

The meaning of touch

The body is covered in sensitive nerve endings and touch is immediate and profound. Health practitioners are privileged to be able to use touch as a form of communication unlike other professions whom we depend on like bankers, lawyers and traders (Tschudin 1999). Nurses and midwives touch more often and more intimately than any of the other professions, and in addition, in personal physical care such as bathing, helping people to mobilise and helping them to eat, the nurse has opportunities for connection and transcendence not open to other professions. It is often during personal physical care that patients confide their fears about losing control and becoming dependent, as well as the time when they talk about their deepest spiritual worries (Picco et al. 2010).

Touch is one of the five senses of human beings and is essential to human life. Yet it is probably the least researched sense and the one scientists have least knowledge about, perhaps because of the complexity of researching such a complex subject. Touch is different in so many ways from other sense organs that scholars have wondered whether it is even comparable. The touch sense organ is the whole body and not just a tiny organ like the eye or ear. Unlike with sight or sound which is carried through the air to the ear or the eye, touch depends on close contact. Touch is also different because when the touch is by a person, that person also feels touched and can be affected emotionally and get feedback from the person they are touching in a much more detailed and profound way than hearing the sound of our own voice or knowing that you are being seen. To be touched means to feel ourselves being touched. Through being touched we not only become aware of something outside of ourselves but we also become more aware of ourselves in contact with the thing that is touching us. In this way a touch may make it more possible for a person to experience being in their own body because a touch brings us back to an awareness of ourselves (van Manen 1999). Supportive touch dissolves the distance between people and restores a sense of being back with yourself, in the world and belonging (van Manen 1999). Suzy Fenton relates how she deliberately used touch to help to restore a young woman's sense of identity when she had a fungating breast tumour.

> I wished to restore Sally's sense of sensuality physical attractiveness, and sexuality. I wanted to make her feel like she was a normal, unimpaired, beautiful person, and I felt that the power of touch would confirm this.
>
> (Fenton 2011, p. 62)

Sensuality is part of our identity and essential for wholeness, so to experience yourself as a sensual and sexual being is something everyone has a right to want to feel until they die regardless of age or infirmity.

Touch impacts on awareness of who we are because it breaches personal boundaries. Because touch breaches our personal space it could threaten our survival, yet it protects us because it allows us to sense pain. It allows aggression and at the same time communicates love and sexuality. Touch is closely linked to the imagination and the feeling of touch becomes embedded in memory so that we can imagine a touch before it happens because the feeling of a touch and the effect it has is remembered within the body. This suggests that the care and valuing and empathy transmitted by a touch could also become embedded in the body and leave a memory of care and love. The modern world makes itself present to us through an increasing array of technological devices rather than by mere bodily experience so that we are increasingly disembodied and treat our bodies more and more as instruments forgetting how much our bodies are capable of remembering, performing and experiencing (Csepregi 2006).

Touch tends to command attention more swiftly and immediately than other senses, perhaps because a provocative or frightening sound could still be at some distance whereas a touch says that someone or something is within our own boundaries. Touch tends to overcome the distance between people more easily than any other sense. With sight or sound the content, what is said or seen is clearer and as important as the tone or the emotion behind it, whereas with touch, the content being transmitted is less clear and response is often on a purely emotional level and therefore in a more direct way than other sensory stimuli.

Touch is the most well-developed sense that humans have at birth and it influences how humans develop throughout childhood and adolescence. If infants are deprived of touch their emotional and mental intelligence is seriously affected (Autton 1989). Touch not only communicates emotions but studies show that the person touched can sense the quality and scale of the emotion communicated with the touch. Touch can also intensify the emotion which is being communicated in the mind of the person being touched. The emotions of anger, fear, disgust, love, gratitude and sympathy can be conveyed by touch even when the subjects in the experiment could not see the faces of those touching (Hertenstein et al. 2006). We use the same language to describe physical touch as we do to describe emotions. When we say we are touched we could mean either a physical hand upon us or that we have been emotionally affected by something. When people describe their emotions they often use the language of physicality; they throb, ache or glow with the intensity of their feelings (Nathan 2007).

When touch is performed with empathy, it can say to the patient that 'I am also like you', 'I can be alongside you in this' and so it reinforces their personhood and dignity. Gadow (1985, p. 41) calls empathic touch 'concern made tangible' because it expresses concern for a person when sometimes words can't. Empathic touch has the ability to create a sense of fellow feeling, to break through into a person's solitude so that they feel less alone. Empathic touch transmits a sense of the value of a person and in so doing could help someone to feel connected to someone or something outside themselves and connected and integrated within themselves. To be prepared to touch someone who is on the margins of society or who has a disease or disability which would normally provoke disgust and withdrawal is an especially valuable gesture of love and compassion. This is recognised in some traditions as an innately spiritual act (Clarke 2011).

From critical care to elderly care, patients have reported that being touched can make them feel more positive towards nurses, it calms and comforts and helps them to cope. For example, in a study with 25 elderly patients in long-term care and their 30 nurses, Routasalo and Isola (1996) found that patients felt the touch of a nurse was warm, gentle and comforting. The patients were aware when a touch was spontaneous and not essential to carry out a particular activity and they especially valued this non-necessary touch, when they felt down and needed their spirits raised.

Touch is received more positively if hands are warm and the touch is relaxed and smooth and if it is accompanied by eye contact and positive sounding speech. If hands are cold and movements are erratic, or if the touch is from someone who is perceived as preoccupied and hurried, feelings about the touch are more likely to be negative (McCabe and Timmins 2006). Patients perceive touch qualitatively, they are not dispassionate about it or indifferent to it. Touch will always invoke a reaction in the person being touched. It also seems to force itself upon our awareness and lead us to make judgements and form opinions about what is being transmitted and about the person who has touched us. It can create a connection, or a disruption in a relationship. Patients identified bad temper as well as kindness by the way they were touched by nurses (Routasalo and Isola 1996).

Many practitioners innately know how to use touch, they know that sometimes an overwrought patient will respond to a touch better than trying to talk to them. Nurses use touch to communicate when a patient has difficulties using words or were worried and they use it to show that they are listening. They also use it to communicate emotions such as liking, loving, caring, sympathy or when they want to be comforting and calming (Routasalo and Isola 1996). Touch is so powerful that touching a person while making a verbal request has been proven to increase the likelihood that the request will be carried out. Researchers have found that if they touch a person lightly while asking them to take part in a survey they are more likely to agree to take part. Touching a patient while saying how important it was to take a particular medication resulted in improved medication compliance (Guéguen and Vion 2009). Skilled practitioners have probably always unconsciously used touch to gain a patient's trust.

In ITUs where patients may be sedated and ventilated, immobile and dependent, touch becomes even more important and always has to be preceded by communication to announce your entry into the patient's space and a careful reading of cues to gauge how any touch will be received. Touch that has been properly heralded and is within a trusting relationship can be a powerful connecting force between the patient and their nurse. One nurse respondent in a study by Estabrooks and Morse (1992, p. 453) called this 'bumping souls'. Nurses who enjoy giving physical care usually learn that it deepens and enhances their relationships with patients and makes their own job more satisfying. Nevertheless nurses vary in the amount of physical contact they want with patients. Sometimes nurses say that they like the kind of care that allows them to use touch, but they don't feel they have time to do as much as they'd like (Picco et al. 2010). However, to patients it tends not to be the amount of time devoted to them that makes the difference, but what the nurse does and what their attitude is during the small moments of time they have together.

The value of being in a closed and intimate situation with someone such as bathing is well known by nurses to help people to open up and talk when they might not otherwise. What might not have been recognised before is the role that touch plays in such situations, bathing and massage have both been shown to encourage confidences to be shared and being in these situations with patients is one way for nurses to help people to talk about their spirituality (Twigg 2000, Taylor 1995).

How to touch: Gentle power

> Nurses are not generally gentle with their clients, in the sense of very soft, delicate touching. Because they are used to the weight of a human body, the toughness of skin, the resistance created by stiffened bones and muscles, they know how to move firmly and strongly. But the very sureness and power of their touch leads to a paradoxical tenderness. The skilled nurse knows that touch needs to be powerful enough to create a sense of security.
>
> (Groenhout et al. 2005, p. 151)

Groenhout et al. describe here the paradox between power and gentleness and how they complement rather than contradict each other. An American nursing tutor described an incident to the scholar van Manen (1999) that happened with a group of nursing students who had been taught to palpate patients' organs and then sent out to a ward full of patients to practice. After a while the tutor noticed that they were holding back and stalling. When she confronted them they gave a string of excuses for their lack of activity, they thought maybe the patients wouldn't want to be bothered, maybe they would have other things to do. When the tutor asked the students to reflect on why they were so reluctant to do the task, a different set of reasons emerged. The students felt that there was such a fine dividing line in perception between, what they called, professional and non-professional touch that they were worried they would do it the wrong way. When the tutor asked them to say what was different in the two types of touch the students said very clearly, 'the professional touch is firm, not light, confident and directed with purpose, goal and intent' (van Manen 1999, p. 7). One student related how she was practising palpation on her sister who had rebuked her for touching her too lightly and suggested that if she touched a patient like that it would be misinterpreted. The story demonstrates that this kind of knowledge is embedded in all of us, but fear of getting it wrong makes us tentative. The patients in O'Lynn and Krautscheid's study (2011) also said, 'Touch me professionally, not too fast and not too slow', 'Touch firmly, not tentative, not caressing', and 'any kind of hesitance would make me feel more anxious and less inclined to let them bathe me' (p. 29). Nurses often pull back from being too firm because they think it might hurt, but actually it is usually what patients want. With firmness, patients also commented on the speed of touch; too quick and it looks like you're embarrassed and trying to get it over as fast as possible but too slow feels lingering which is uncomfortable.

Thinking time

Stop and think for a few minutes about how you feel about touching someone when you're caring for them.

Ask yourself whether you touch as much as possible or as little as possible.

Do you try to avoid touching?

If you have any fears or worries about touching, stop and think about what they are and what might make you feel differently.

Cultural and personal differences

It has been argued that in the Western world there is a taboo about touch and an epidemic of injunctions against touch, as if a natural caution has grown into a fear of being touched and a disproportionate awareness of personal boundaries; perhaps because of an excessive association between touch and sex which is apparently an English disease (Autton 1989). Whatever the reason, generally in the West, it has come to be normal to see touch as something dangerous and risky and less social touching takes place in the United States and Western Europe than in other parts of the world (Argyle 1988) with injunctions against adults touching children being particularly strong. In terms of purely expressive touching, the stroke on an arm or a hug can be disempowering when it is used to dominate (Argyle 1988, Routasalo and Isola 1996). Health care is aimed at empowerment yet it is unavoidably true that patients do have to depend upon practitioners for physical help and for their knowledge. Practitioners make decisions about patient's lives which inevitably make for relationships which have innate power imbalances and the practitioner needs to be aware of this and always try to redress the balance in favour of the patient. Because people don't give everyone permission to touch them, those who assume the power to touch are always in a dominant position and a patient can feel as though they are being denied the power to refuse. Touching can be experienced as an act of domination, especially when it takes place between people who don't know each other (Routasalo and Isola 1996). For instance, one common way of asserting superiority over someone in certain contexts is to put a hand on their shoulder. Women often experience this as patronising when it comes from domineering men (Argyle 1988) who are standing above them. It can be difficult to measure when a touch might appear this way but being on the same physical level as someone helps; as does greeting them and introducing yourself first; making eye contact, and feeling genuine concern. However, although the occasion may not be right for a deliberate expressive touch, that doesn't mean that instrumental touching, whilst taking a temperature or helping someone to stand, can't also express concern, care, empathy, patience, warmth and the confirmation of personhood. As has been discussed in the previous chapter, attention is expressed in the body, as long as it is believed in by the practitioner. Patients can sense the emotion and intent behind a touch, so that practitioners have be clear in their own minds what their intentions are.

Example

When I was a student nurse a clinical tutor arrived on the ward one morning to work with me. I was about to bed bath a man and I turned to get something from his locker and out of the corner of my eye I saw the tutor standing at the end of the bed speaking to the patient asking him how long he'd been in hospital and how he felt, just routine chat. But as she did so she had her hands on his lower legs which were uncovered and was gently moving her hands up and down over his shins stroking his skin. I felt the man melt and relax before I even turned to look at him. He looked so appreciative, calm and somehow stronger than I'd seen him before. I was struck by how such a simple act could have such an effect. I thought even back then as a student, what an amazing gift a nurse could give just by such simple acts of kindness.

Touching as in the example above was acceptable in that context. If a relative was present it would not have been appropriate; in an outpatient clinic, it would not be appropriate; if she had not spoken to the patient first and introduced herself, it would not be appropriate; if she had not also been talking to the patient, it would not have been appropriate; if she had not been wearing a uniform and a badge, it would not have been appropriate; if there had been the slightest sign from the patient that it was unwelcome, I am sure she would not have continued for an instant.

While there are no cultures where touch is completely prohibited (Argyle 1988) as has been stated earlier, some cultures use touch more than others, in Arab countries more and in the United Kingdom, United States and the West in general less. People in France and southern Europe touch more than those in the north (Field 1999, Twigg 2000). However, most studies have been in social settings not care settings and in general most people accept touch when it is from a professional wearing a uniform and name badge in a caring setting and when the context and occasion feels right. Touch is inappropriate when it is given at the wrong time, in the wrong dose or to the wrong person (Autton 1989).

Cuing for touch

Nurses who are used to using touch as part of their relationship with patients often use their intuition and experience to discern signs or cues such as facial expression, eye contact and body movements to tell whether patients are open to being touched (Estabrooks and Morse 1992). The first time you meet a patient is often a key time to gauge how much touch and how much emotional contact they want (Picco et al. 2010). Patients are aware that they use non-verbal signs to signal that they would be open to 'being patted'; sometimes this was just in a look towards the nurse (Routasalo and Isola's 1996). Banning all non-necessary touch without express permission is a policy born out of fear and it detracts from the spontaneity of a natural and compassionate act (Bates 2007), but there is a need for judgement to choose the right place, with the right person and the right amount. Sometimes nurses sense that the right touch is a hug and students seem also to see this but report that they rarely see patients touched just for comfort in practice (Hardy 2011). If nurses are expected to interact with wholeness they should not be denied the freedom to use their own judgement.

The traditional way of approaching a person in the West has been to shake hands, a gesture which has to some extent gone into disuse in recent decades probably because it came to be associated with a stiff formality. However, the alternative, a hug is not appropriate when you have just met someone, so perhaps it is time to bring back the handshake. A handshake is universally understood as being a gesture of welcome and peace and friendliness. It gives an initial and non-threatening touch approach to a patient and it can allow the nurse to learn something about a patient just from the feel of their hand. It can be as formal or as warm as the situation seems to need and it can be modified to include the opposite hand also resting on the other's hand. It should always be accompanied by the attempt to make eye contact.

Using touch in mental health nursing

Mental illness can cause people to be particularly sensitive to any encroachment on their person or personal space and so it is not surprising to find that mental health nurses use touch less than other groups (Gleeson and Higgins 2009), to the extent that there has been a powerful embargo on touch in mental health practice which some mental health practitioners believe is unwarranted (Autton 1989). In fact today many mental health nurses see touch as a useful and potent tool especially if it is used expressively and not just as part of procedures (Gleeson and Higgins 2009). Nurses felt it was therapeutic not only for the comfort it could provide but also because it helped to disperse the barriers between nurse and patient, helping patients to open up more. One nurse said that they would nearly always shake hands when they first met a client and this helped them to develop a rapport. These nurses used touch to reinforce something that they were saying verbally, to give reassurance and to express how they cared for someone. They felt that what you expressed by touching someone would be seen as more sincere and more heartfelt than what you said, so that if you really wanted to get through to someone you touched them. If you said 'well done' that was okay, but a pat on the shoulder at the same time would mean more to the client. Touch was also used when words were inadequate and more reassurance was required, or when clients didn't want to talk and silence was the most appropriate response but with the reassurance that you were there (Gleeson and Higgins 2009).

> When somebody is very depressed they've lost all hope, they're in complete bleakness, they feel very isolated and alone . . . so I'd touch them on the arm.
> (Gleeson and Higgins 2009, p. 386)

As in other specialities mental health nurses assessed cues, by using light touches at first and assessing mood and atmosphere. They used what they knew about patients to help them make judgements about using touch. They valued touch and felt it was important to use it. Men in particular felt they needed to use caution so as not to provoke allegations of sexual attention (Gleeson and Higgins 2009). Mixed sex teams need to talk about these issues and explore ways that the problems might be overcome so that female patients are not disadvantaged when cared for by male staff. For instance, by using touch in public but not in private; or by focusing attention and warmth into a handshake or eye contact.

Conclusion

In this chapter we have seen the possibilities of touch for forming relationships and enabling integration and wholeness. Touch is a powerful tool which nurses and midwives can use to affect the spiritual well-being of patients and we should not be afraid to use it as long as we use judgment and discernment. The remaining three chapters will look in detail at the spiritual disintegration that occurs as people become more dependent on others for help with meeting the essentials of life, like moving, bathing and eating. What we have learnt so far about relationships, caring, comfort, body and touch will come together in how we help people to move, bathe and eat.

12 Helping people to move

Introduction

Helping people to move is one of the most common things that nurses do. From helping someone to sit up in bed, to moving from bed to chair, to sitting on a toilet and helping someone to regain their walking skills; it is a constant task. Midwives move people into the best position for birthing and mental health nurses coax people around corridors and bathrooms or in and out of beds.

It is a prime opportunity to show care and encouragement through the manipulation of their physical body using touch. This chapter will take a detailed look at what happens between patient and nurse in the nursing act to unpick what the nurse can do to make the care they give endorse and strengthen the patient's spiritual well-being. At the end, a table will link all the things you can do to the effects they might have spiritually.

The moving dance of care: Spirituality in moving

The spiritual care in helping people to move rests in finding a balance between providing security while at the same time encouraging the patient to find their own power and take control so that in this way they are not diminished by accepting help and are enabled to experience their body as less of a hindrance. This means you, as the nurse, have to relinquish control, which involves some sacrifice of professional power. It is also an opportunity to be caring and to demonstrate that you respect and value the person you are helping. As in all these acts of care, you begin to affect the patient's spirituality as soon as you approach them by involving them in planning the move, valuing their ideas and protecting their modesty. Making conversation brings the patient into the flow of life and makes them feel included. You can communicate compassion through how you touch both instrumentally when providing security and instruction and expressively when giving encouragement and expressing solidarity and empathy. In the act of helping a patient from bed to chair, nurse and patient manoeuvre around each other, the patient's weight shifting, the feet shuffling as the patient shifts and moves to stay in balance with the nurse (Groenhout et al. 2005). Patients rarely want the nurse to bear their whole weight, they want to help and they know that too much help, like too much weight, can put the nurse at risk. There is a delicate balance to be achieved. The extent to which the patient resists or cooperates is a reflection of the relationship the nurse and patient have managed to achieve between them. The decision by the patient to accept assistance may seem a small one, but to a patient their whole life may be bound up in it and it presents a panoply of questions. How independent can I be? If I accept now that I can't get out of bed without help, is that a temporary blip or the way it's always going to be? Is this a time when I should summon my courage and determination and say no, stand back I'll do this alone, or is it a time when I should give you permission to help (when in fact I'm going to try with all my might to do it without leaning on you, even if that means that I pull you down with me). Nurses have all said at some time to a patient, 'just let yourself go floppy'. Meaning, it will really be better if you just let *me* do this. For a patient that means total dependence which not only requires a high degree of trust, but could herald the realisation that they will never be independent again. Groenhout et al. (2005, p. 151) call this shifting of weight and balance, the steps of which have to be learnt by both parties, a 'dance'. Patients want to feel they are in secure, confident hands when they are being cared for (Groenhout et al. 2005, p. 151, O'Lynn and Krautscheid 2011) but they also want to stand alone. Competence and confidence can be conveyed by the balance of tenderness and firmness. De Hennezel (1998) describes the rhythm created by two nurses together, caring for one patient in a hospice:

> whenever they (*nurse's aides*) go to give whatever body assistance is required by someone who can no longer even move in bed, they are aware of how much the fact of being there for each other and of bringing the patient into this link creates a completely different kind of contact. The movements they so gently make to lift a leg and ease a patient over onto his

side synchronise themselves of one accord and flow together without jolts or bumping. When one cleans a bedsore, the other embraces the enfeebled body and just stays there doing nothing but rocking it gently.

(De Hennezel 1998, p. 50)

As this situation describes, this is valuable time with a patient when tasks are carried out but within it tenderness and value are transmitted. Technical skill alone is not enough to give care which affects the spirit, yet care without technical skill is also not enough. Valuing the person and their welfare is the professional love which adds care to skill and this will be demonstrated if the nurse chooses it. Empathy in the physical act of helping someone to move is in the sensing of what will cause pain and how it can be avoided. Ask most expert nurses if they can sense pain in someone else and know where it is and how they can avoid it and they may say no. But watch them help someone in pain to move and it is clear that empathy is enabling them in each moment to sense exactly where the pain is and where to place their hands. It is during moments of concentrated skilled care that complete empathic presence with another person is possible in otherwise hectic days, flying from one task to another.

> Thus, the caring hand that gently supports a patient as she turns to find a new position in bed does not touch the skin which encloses a body, but this hand touches the woman herself. The gentle contact of the hand and the woman's body is a direct contact between two human beings, the nurse 'with' the patient. We notice that the caring hand anticipates the pain involved in moving, slips so easily under us, fitting perfectly to the curvatures of our back, and finding just the right place to support us. The fear of pain vanishes for a moment as we both move together to a new position with ease. From this place, the world takes on a different light. Yet, there is some ambiguity here, for even a patient knows that simple procedures, like repositioning someone in bed, have a skillful element. Perhaps, when procedures are accomplished with the skillful hand alone, the patient is not comforted. Perhaps, it is only the caring hand that comforts.

(Bottorff 1991, p. 247)

Here Bottorf captures the almost unconscious knowledge that an expert nurse has of how and where to support a person to move and the fact that for comfort to happen neither technical skill nor care alone are enough but both have to be brought together.

Thinking time

Think back to the last time you helped someone to move. What were you thinking about while you did it? Reflect on what you were wanting to achieve when you did it. Was it just about helping them to move? Could you have been aiming to do more?

The spiritual care in helping a patient to move

Action	Spiritual rationale
• Include the patient in planning what is going to happen and deciding the aims. • Invite the patient to make as many of the decisions as possible. • Give as many choices as possible. • Explain any mobility equipment and the reasons for its use.	• Empowers the patient and reinforces their personhood. • Shows that you see them as a person as valid in the world as yourself. • Respects their wishes and so values them as a person. • Makes the patient feel cared for because you are interested in them.
• Find out what the patient wants to do for themselves and include as much patient activity as possible.	• Shows that you see them as still having an essential contribution to make.
• Use your presence – Give your whole attention to the patient. • Make eyes contact.	• Helps the patient to feel loved, cared for and accepted because they are worthy of your focused attention.
• Be patient, allowing time for the patient to act independently as much as possible.	• Helps the patient to feel included in the flow of life, shows that their way of doing things is as valid and valuable as your own.

(Continued)

Action	Spiritual rationale
• Use firm and gentle touch where holding and balancing is necessary.	• Makes the patient feel secure and cared for. • Makes them feel accepted as a person who can be touched.
• Talk to the patient during, before and after the activity.	• Demonstrates that you are interested in the person. • Chat about non-nursing things includes them in the flow of life. • Shows empathy and compassion.
• Sense where the weight of the patient is balanced and co-ordinate with it.	• Shows ability to act in partnership with the patient and not take control.

Conclusion

Being able to move independently is fundamental to being a person and so needing help is an immediately disempowering situation to be in, which you can help to alleviate by your care.

13 Helping people to bathe

Introduction

De Hennezel describes below, in talking about the care of one patient, how the potentially humiliating experience of being bathed by another can be transformed to not only being bearable but actually dignity enhancing and so self-enhancing, by helping the patient to feel valued, whole and cared for, by in fact restoring his humanity.

> By choosing to clean him with affection, so that he can experience the fact that even when he's soiled, he's still worthy of my greatest care and attention, I have perhaps repaired his feeling of being nothing but human scrap, something rather dirty. This acknowledgment of his fundamental humanity is balm on the wound inflicted by insult.
>
> (De Hennezel 1998, p. 116)

In this chapter the act of bathing someone else will be explored to see how it can be made something which can contribute to a person's spiritual well-being by the way it is performed. A summary at the end will link what you do to the spiritual effects it could have.

Bathing and caring: Spiritual care in the bed bath

This is challenging work because the power imbalances inherent between patients and nurses are accentuated when the patient is supine, half naked and dependent and the nurse stands and is clothed and there to help. Van Manen relates the experience related to him of one man who was recovering from a heart problem which shows how these experiences stay in the mind, long after you are well.

The nurse was washing me, stroking, scrubbing and refreshing my sore and tired body in a way that I experienced as extremely agreeable and consoling – yet there was not a hint of arousal in the experience. I remember that the nurse talked to me all the while she washed my body, although I was too foggy to now remember what she said and what I may have said. It does not matter. I just remember the bathing. How I simply felt so much better, physically better in a way that was indeed experienced as healing. That is the best word I have for it, 'physical healing'. The nurse touching me had a peculiar effect: I was allowed to be myself and to feel my own body again.

(van Manen 1998, p. 2)

This man quite unexpectedly experiences more than simply being made clean. The combination of touch, care and the experience of being bathed feels innately healing to him. As though another stage on the way to recovery is accomplished, body and soul are brought back together again.

Twigg's research with carers and patients about their experiences of being bathed found that what they thought most horrifying is to be bathed by someone who they suspect finds it repulsive so that they would prefer to go unwashed than be washed by someone doing it unwillingly (Twigg 2000). As one participant said, 'She thought it was absolutely disgusting . . . you felt she is doing you such a favour, you prefer not to – you prefer to stink actually' (Twigg 2000, p. 56).

O'Lynn and Krautscheid (2011) sought the views of 24 patients about what they wanted from nurses when they were receiving intimate personal care, and found that patients wanted to have plenty of communication before the care was given which included some explanation about what was to happen. Patients said that they especially wanted to have some communication with nurses before any kind of intimate touch took place; they wanted to feel that they had a relationship with the nurse who was to bathe them, 'a human connection', said one patient (O'Lynn and Krautscheid 2011, p. 27). Humour helped some people to overcome their embarrassment and silence could be uncomfortable.

They appreciated it if the nurse imparted some information about themselves. Yet at the same time as wanting to have a warm and friendly relationship with the nurse they also wanted an element of professional distance and so they thought their nurse should be presented professionally with a clean and tidy uniform. These patients wanted to be given choices, and this meant besides having some explanation about what was to take place, they wanted to decide for themselves whether they needed help or not and especially whether they needed help with washing very private parts of their body. The patients in O'Lynn's and Krautscheid's study (2011) expressed how 'powerless and devalued' they felt when they weren't able to decide things for themselves about intimate care. 'They treated me like a two year old', said one woman, 'it was almost like I wasn't there', said another (2003, p. 28). The patients in a study by Routasalo and Isola (1996) wanted to be greeted before being touched and they wanted to be touched without gloves whenever possible as gloves were considered emotionally cold, but interestingly, the nurses in the same study seemed to think that the patients hadn't noticed the gloves (Routasola and Isola 1996). Communication in situations which are potentially embarrassing or intimate is not just a way to get information from patients but it also oils the wheels of relationship, it enables trust to develop and it shows warm humanity. Asking about choices makes people feel that you value their contribution and you take it for granted that they will have opinions about how they want to wash, what products they want to use and what clothes they want to wear. This makes people feel valued and helps to make someone feel 'normal'. These are the choices that ordinary people make, people who are not ill, not old, not disabled, and they are the choices that I can still make. While patients vary about the importance of the gender of the nurse giving intimate care, many people want to choose the gender of the person giving them help with bathing, no matter what their age or disability. It is a fact that while it is accepted that women can bathe men and women, women often only want to be bathed by other women. In addition, some men prefer to be bathed by a woman, as women are considered more neutral gendered because of their maternal links, and it avoids possible undertones of homosexuality (Twigg 2000, O'Lynn and Krautscheid 2011). Health professionals have to try to accommodate wishes about gender and usually providers of care accept this as a very deep-rooted choice. It is not uncommon for female patients even of a great age, where it is tempting to think that it can be ignored, to refuse bathing rather than be bathed by a man. If these kinds of deep cultural requirements are ignored a person can easily start to feel devalued and it can begin to erode their personhood. It is especially insidious where cultural norms about gender are cast aside for older people but not for younger.

Thinking time

Think about the last time you had a bath or a shower.

Take a few minutes to think about how it would feel to have someone else do all the same things for you, another person who you had never met.

How do you think you would feel?

How would you like them to be towards you?

Most often when patients feel no embarrassment or shame in these situations it is because they have never felt embarrassed to be naked and this is an aspect of their personality. However, it may also be that they have been forced to condition themselves not to care anymore (Twigg 2000, O'Lynn and Krautscheid 2011). Most people have some degree of embarrassment in being naked in front of someone else and when staff declare that they've seen it all and are not concerned, that doesn't make any difference. One patient said, 'I know like they all say, Oh, if I've seen one body, I've seen them all, ... but not *me*, ... and it doesn't make you feel any better them saying that' (Twigg 2000, p. 56).

Helping someone to maintain their identity and sense of selfhood and feel whole is more likely to be achieved by accepting them as the person they are, with their embarrassment, rather than expecting and coaxing them to be a different sort of person who is not embarrassed to be naked. Sometimes embarrassment is exacerbated by nurses who appear as passive observers, viewing a spectacle, rather than active helpers. One patient said of a nurse who was 'supervising' her shower, 'Don't just stand there and watch me bathe. Help or get out!' (O'Lynn and Krautscheid 2011, p. 29).

Being willing to disclose something about yourself such as your hobbies and interests helps to disperse embarrassment. It also makes you into a human being and shows that you trust and like the person you are caring for, and so they are more likely to trust and like you. Knowing the person who is helping you in intimate tasks is very important, which is why greeting someone and talking to them before the task is so crucial. Shame and embarrassment at being naked affects everyone regardless of age, to the point that patients will refuse bathing when their usual carer is on holiday, rather than be bathed by a stranger (Twigg 2000). This is particularly difficult when you are in a team with many staff. Patients naturally feel annoyed when they have to contend with a completely new person to go through the embarrassment of exposure with, when the person who helped them the day before is allocated to the patient next to them. So that as far as is possible, there should be continuity in nurses and if that can't be achieved, a patient deserves some explanation about why staff have to be changed.

In Twigg's (2000, p. 59) study both patients and carers emphasised the back as a site where touch could be neutral and it could be vigorous and comforting. If the nurse is at the back of the patient the vulnerable and private parts are covered. Similarly an arm across the back provides non-threatening comfort.

Privacy is essential to a person's sense of self-worth and this means having closed doors and their own bodies exposed as little as possible. Patients particularly don't like gowns and blankets that aren't secured properly (O'Lynn and Krautscheid 2011). When something embarrassing is happening talk and humour can help to divert attention and normalise the situation.

The spiritual care in helping a patient to bathe

Action	Spiritual rationale
• Introduce yourself (wear a name badge). • Talk (perhaps about something not related to the task); say something about yourself and use humour. • Shake hands or use touch to make contact. • Make eye contact.	• Demonstrates respect, adds the balance of professional distance. • Helps to allay embarrassment. • Establishes a relationship • Establishes you as someone who can be trusted. • Shows warmth, humanity and compassion.

(Continued)

Action	Spiritual rationale
• Find out about the person you are helping. • Ask questions to discover their wishes and any preferences. • Give as many choices as possible. • Show awareness of any cultural or personal preferences if you know them or interest and curiosity if you don't. • Plan as much as possible with the patient, or ask them what their plan is. • Explain what will happen and check with them that they agree with the plan.	• Empowers and shows you value their help and opinion. • Shows that you see them as a person as valid in the world as yourself. • Self-esteem is increased if you feel someone is interested in you. • Shows respect.
• Give your whole attention to the patient while you are helping them. • Use your presence, make frequent eye contact.	• Helps the patient to feel loved, cared for and accepted because they are worthy of your focused attention. • Attention which is focused but not intense when an activity is happening can allow the person to talk without feeling too much of the spotlight on them. They may talk about spiritual concerns they wouldn't say in another situation.
• Gather together everything needed, including the patient's wishes. • Make sure water is at the right temperature	• Shows that you care and value the patient's contribution.
• Touch firmly and swiftly but not hurriedly • Only wear gloves where necessary according to the infection control policy.	• Makes the patient feel secure and accepted. • Massage soothes and relaxes and makes someone feel cared for, accepted and whole.

- Include massage and rubs, if you feel prepared and confident, only when the patient is not uncovered completely and only with their permission.

- Being touched with care and having confidence in the nurse could help the patient to relax and allow themselves to be in someone else's hands. This may help them to transcend in their mind the current situation, feeling whole again.

- Use conversation to show interest in the patient and to relieve embarrassment.
- Talk about other things rather than the task

- Shows sensitivity to the person's feelings.
- Talking about life outside the hospital or home helps the person to feel included in the flow of life. Shows that you value the person and their life.
- Shows you are interested in the person and helps to make the patient feel cared for.

- Only uncover as much of the patient as is absolutely necessary.
- Make sure doors and curtains are secure.
- Don't allow interruptions.

- Shows respect and empathy

Conclusion

Bathing is one of the most intimate acts we do for ourselves and when someone else is helping it can leave a person feeling invaded, disempowered, infantilised and exposed. How the nurse manages the situation and performs the task has the potential to provide comfort which enhances self-esteem, provide connection and restore dignity and humanity.

14 Helping people to eat

Introduction

Eating is not only an activity that we closely identify with independent living, but it is also essential to survival and is loaded with cultural, social, ethical, religious and moral significance (Gastmans 1998). To be unable to eat independently is a huge blow to selfhood and self-esteem. Depending on someone else to give you food or help you eat is disempowering and sensitive and spiritual care can enable someone to regain some control over this area of their life. This chapter will look at how nurses provide food at mealtimes to all patients and how they help people who need assistance to eat.

Providing food and assisted eating: The spirituality of food in nursing

Eating is bound up with social rules and personal preferences. A meal is not just about eating to live, it is expected to be a pleasurable event and it is often central to the day. It is most often a social event; it helps people to form and confirm connections and relationships, it brings people together and cements family life. Food and eating marks cultural and religious commemorations, celebrations, feasts and rites of passage; the food we eat marks the passage of time, most people still eat with the seasons to some extent. How and what we eat expresses our identity; it confirms our similarities with each other and our uniqueness (Perry 2008). Eating is also related to hospitality; food is offered in every culture to make others feel at ease, relaxed and comfortable. Most people can talk at length about the food they like and don't like; their memory of particular meals; their cooking skills or lack of them; their choice of restaurants; and their expectations of guests at meals. Therefore any disturbance to the ability to offer or receive hospitality choose the food we eat and to eat it independently is usually painful and disturbing. It can be a blow to selfhood and self-esteem and anything that the nurse can do to restore choice and independence will contribute to restoring wholeness, identity and the ability to connect with the world again. Lifting some of the burden of anxiety around the getting and eating of food can strengthen personhood, providing confirmation and confidence so that the patient can focus on recovery, or enable them to recover identity and selfhood to be able to accept and manage long-term dependence.

Showing sensitivity to worries and preferences around food demonstrates compassionate care. Ensuring that someone is well fed is highly symbolic of care and hospitality and so solving eating-related problems and ensuring that the process of eating is relaxed and dignified is one of the most important nursing acts.

As sickness and disability bring a more sedentary lifestyle and isolation, meals can take on even more significance and to be unable to eat what and how you want is depressing. Food may begin to matter less and the appetite wanes so restricting recovery. One of the biggest complaints that patients and their relatives make about care whilst in hospital revolves around food. Problems include malnutrition because nurses have not ensured that patients had enough food to eat, providing food that patients couldn't reach or manage or which was inedible, or giving inadequate help so that patients felt a loss of dignity. Incidents such as these more often seem to affect older people in hospitals and they affect their families and friends who have to look on powerless (Age UK 2010, The Patients Association 2011). These examples from patients and relatives are typical.

I noticed two other patients being given their lunch and left alone, before their uneaten lunch was just taken away from them. Nobody asked whether they wanted or needed any help.
(The Patients Association 2011, p. 24)

She had food all down her chin from the last meal that she had eaten.

(p. 67)

Very often the meals would be cold by the time the patients were sat up, meaning that they became even more inedible than they have started out. The pureed food offered to these patients was abysmal. I had to take in food every day for mum.

(p. 68)

Angela and Sally also witnessed their mother, and several other patients, being left without food because they could not manage to eat on their own, for example carrying out a simple task such as opening a sandwich packet.

(p. 69)

The nurses' role in bringing assisted eating into the realm of spiritual care is in helping people who need help with eating to avoid feeling excluded and infantilised and to restore dignity and personhood. The nurse is trying as much as possible to reproduce what the person would want for themselves.

There are social rules about eating such as food must be put cleanly and quietly into the mouth in the right amounts. Dribbling and opening the mouth with food in it are taboos which are considered disgusting and people who eat like this risk rejection. Being able to follow the rules and eat cleanly without drawing attention to oneself is a sign of maturity and enables us to fit in socially, and to be unable to do it yourself is instantly felt as a return to a childlike dependent state.

People who have had a stroke say that being unable to eat what they want independently caused a severe sense that the person they had been was lost. They could no longer present themselves to others in the way they wanted to, and this led to embarrassment and shame which led to isolation as social and family activities were curtailed. Foods which had been loved and which were a part of their personality were suddenly off limits, usually because they were just too difficult to eat and they were embarrassed and ashamed of eating in public (Perry and McLaren 2003).

People lose their ability to eat independently for many reasons and there are now a range of therapeutic interventions for patients that need assistance from intravenous or Percutaneous Endoscopic Gatrostomy (PEG) feeds to simply helping someone to cut up their food and many stages in-between. The next section will focus on helping you to see the spiritual aspects of assisting people to eat in a way that can be applied to all situations, focusing on mealtimes and assisted eating.

Mealtimes

The expression 'sensitive cooperation' which was coined by Martinsen et al. (2009) to refer to the completely dependent patient could equally refer to the kind of relationship that nurses need to develop with anyone who needs any degree of help with eating. Whatever degree of help is needed, the nurse has to be sensitive and thoughtful to co-operate with the person who needs help to achieve a good outcome. When people who need help feel forgotten or ignored this leads to feelings of powerlessness (Martinsen et al. 2008). To be kept waiting or forgotten in any situation makes you feel small and insignificant, but when it is in relation to getting food, this is likely to be multiplied. There is an inbuilt antagonism in human beings towards having to ask for help, so to have to ask for help with food is particularly demeaning. To be left mid-way through a meal while your helper goes to do another task adds insult to injury. Therefore mealtimes are opportunities to demonstrate care and central to mealtime management is respect for personhood (Reimer and Keller 2009).

Thoughtful consideration of each stage of the mealtime process is needed, from offering help to choose from a menu and careful assessment to identify likely problems to considering the position you should be in when helping. Standing over someone increases their sense of powerlessness and being fed by someone wearing gloves can make you feel that helping you eat is repulsive.

In recent years it has come to light that elderly people can suffer from malnutrition in their own homes when they can't manage to get or prepare food or just lose their appetite and nobody notices. When people are ill they become catabolic and need even more calories to recover but even in hospital they can lose weight and become undernourished because in a health-care system which is increasingly focused on technology, non-technological simple needs become neglected. This is especially so with elderly people who may be confused, too sick to be bothered eating, can't reach their food or find it too unpalatable to eat.

Personal and spiritual beliefs proliferate where eating and meals are concerned, and respect and understanding for those beliefs denotes respect for the individuals who hold them as well as making it more likely that they will eat. Religions all have rituals about fasting and there are often prayers associated with eating; asking people about these preferences and giving opportunities for prayer show respect for the individual and raises self-esteem. Mealtimes may be occasions when people can be helped to reconnect with the philosophical or religious contexts which give their life meaning by choosing particular foods or by using prayers or preparation rituals (Gastmans 1998). Preparing for mealtimes is part of the ritual of eating, reminding people of the food they have ordered provokes anticipation increasing appetite and most people would like to feel clean and prepared for eating, which also tends to increase appetite.

When textbooks and nurses' language reduces the pleasurable act of eating to procedures for 'nutrition and hydration' instead of 'food and drink', this will tend to translate into practices that are just about improving calorie intake (Reimer and Keller 2009). Whereas seeing the provision of food as hospitality and the creation of environments fits for eating as holistic and part of interpersonal care is more humane. Seeing the provision of food and drink as attending to the whole person as a physical and spiritual entity is more likely to not only improve appetite, but also enable the person to be self-motivated and stronger physically and spiritually. Food has to be attractive and inviting, and it is in this respect that the polarity between patient and nurse is most apparent because nurses frequently put food before patients which they admit they would not eat themselves. It is as if the patient has ceased to become a person and become a different being. Even sieved or pureed food can still be served as separate items and creativity is called for in finding ways to make mealtimes relaxed and enjoyable occasions.

Example

I work on a big ward where lots of people needed help in eating. For years we had a problem of pureed food arriving from the kitchen combined, so that peas, mince and potatoes came as a brown splodge. And we never had time to give the proper attention to the people that needed help, because all the food would arrive at once. We put up with this because we were always told that nothing could be done. It felt like there was this chasm between the ward and the people who supplied the food and we all believed that nothing would get the other side to shift. Then we had a new ward sister who saw the problem, went to the Food Services Manager and instead of making demands, just asked for his help and suggestions in making life better for the patients. He said, 'Oh yes we can do something about that, nobody has ever asked before'. Within a week all the pureed food was coming to the wards in separate parts. We worked out a system for marking the menus of patients who needed help with eating so that by the following week, their food came first and we could focus on them. The rest of the food came in a separate trolley later. Now the Food Manager comes around the wards and talks to the patients and staff to find out what they think of the food and to see if there are any more problems he can solve. He says he loves being involved. We've made other little adjustments like closing the ward door so there's no draught and nobody walking through. We also decide in the morning who will be feeding the patients who need help and they go to lunch early so they're well fed and relaxed before they start.

One of the obstacles to being able to give the right level of help to all who need it has always been insufficient staff and the competing demands in hospitals at mealtimes. To answer this problem the NHS have campaigned for trusts to adopt a policy of protected mealtimes. This means that everyone in the hospital has a responsibility to stay away from wards during meals and no nurses are at lunch so that the maximum number of staff is available to help with eating. This is accompanied by patients being prepared for eating by positioning, tidying up bed areas and hand washing prior to food arriving (National Patient Safety Agency 2007). But for strategies like this to work, nurses have to be prepared to challenge doctors and other therapists who visit patients during meals and ask them to wait.

The very act of eating is spiritual in many cultures and traditions which is reflected in the value people give it, so for nurses to give it value shows respect and value for the individual and helps them to feel relaxed, whole, cared for and connected to the rest of life.

The spiritual care in managing mealtimes

Action	Spiritual rationale
• Prior to the mealtime patients should be invited to choose the food they will eat. • Familiarise yourself with the assessments of the patients in your care.	• Empowers the patient and shows respect for their personhood. • Shows competence and professionalism which expresses care and valuing of patients. • Empowering and shows you value their contribution.

(Continued)

Action	Spiritual rationale
• Invite people who might need assistance to work out a plan including their family and carers for the help they need so that everyone knows what will happen when the food arrives. • There should be choices available which are compatible with the patients' personal, cultural and religious needs.	• Relieves the anxiety in patients of worrying if food will be okay and whether they will be able to eat it. So that patients can feel more relaxed and focus their energy on getting well. • Shows you are sensitive to their individuality and religious and cultural preferences, so recognising patients as full members of the community.
• Make patients comfortable and ready for eating. Give the chance to wash hands and face ready for eating. • Give the option of sitting away from their bed and with other people if possible. • Tidy the area around each patient removing urine bottles and wiping surfaces.	• Shows sensitivity to and respect for patient's feelings. • Shows competence and attention to detail and so inspires trust • Shows how you value the eating experience.
• Check the food is appropriate, attractive, the right temperature and prepared so that each person can manage it. • Ensure it is what the patients ordered.	• Expresses care for the patient and shows that they are valuable enough for you to care if they are not enjoying the food.
• Give help to each person individually without interruption. • Ensure the patient is not disturbed while they eat. • Monitor what food is eaten and how patients' managing where appropriate.	• Expresses care for the patients' needs and concern for their recovery.
• Be prepared to be an advocate for patients to make complaints and make changes if the food is unacceptable or the amount of help available is not enough. • Be imaginative and creative in finding better ways to manage mealtimes.	• Shows the patient that they matter and are valued.

> **Time to think**
>
> Think about all the food you like to eat, the restaurants and café's you like to go to, the social events that revolve around meals, the pleasure you get from snacks during the day. Think about the amount of time you spend making choices, at home, in shops, cafes and bars about what to eat and drink.
>
> Now imagine what it would be like to only be able to eat what someone else gave you, at the speed they chose, in the way they chose in the place they chose.
>
> How do you think you would feel?

Assisting someone to eat

When someone needs help with the actual act of eating, you need to cooperate with the patient, working together to achieve an experience which is as close to what the patient would experience if they were able to eat unaided and as close as possible to what everyone else is experiencing. As eating is such a social activity and is so charged with social and cultural rules, the nurse has to be responsive not only to the patient themselves, but to anyone else in the room and to the patient's family and friends who may be present.

Martinsen et al. (2008) interviewed 16 people who had spinal cord injury and observed them being fed, to learn about the experience of being permanently dependent on being fed by others. They said that that the ideal is for the person helping to exactly reproduce what they themselves would have done. Consequently the person being fed has to feel sure that the person helping them was not only a willing partner who sincerely wants to help but also that they would 'obey' even their smallest wish. The word 'obey' might sound extreme but in this context it is apt because the person being helped, in Martinsen et al.'s words,

> borrows the helper's body to eat and drink and gradually *teaches* [my italics] the other body to follow a new eating pattern.
>
> (Martinsen et al. 2009, p. 710)

Thus you have to be able to lend your body to the patient and allow yourself to be led (and taught) by the person you are helping. Patients who needed complete help described how an eating pattern which was embedded unconsciously in their own body had to be made conscious and taught to someone else to be performed by their (the helper's) body. Helpers need to have sensitivity, empathy and a genuine concern to help someone else: technical expertise alone won't be enough and it will be detected (Martinsen et al. 2009). People who need help with something that used to be unconscious don't necessarily want to have to keep talking about it which may be one reason why sometimes nurses experience irritation in someone they are trying to help. For the nurse this is an occasional activity, for the person being helped, it is a constant effort to have to keep explaining. Some people gave constant directions, 'It's my life. I have to eat how I want', while others had given up,

> It's easier not to say anything. If you start giving directions you are forced into a dialogue about the procedure and I don't like that. I'd rather eat it the way it is done and talk about other things.
>
> (Martinsen et al. 2009, p. 711)

Knowledge of someone else's needs and wishes builds up over time but for a person in a more temporary or acute situation, all the same things apply but there is little time to learn and so there needs to be instant trust between the patient and the nurse and as far as possible some continuity, so the person being helped is not having to repeatedly teach different members of staff. The nurse is the patient's hands, and sometimes, where the patient might have sensory problems, the patient's eyes and nose as well. So the nurse has to put aside her own likes and dislikes and focus on the patient. However, there are some common standards with regard to food and nurses should only offer patients food that they would find acceptable themselves.

The aim of feeding someone should be 'normality'. Being dependent on someone else to eat can be a very humiliating experience and so everything should be done to minimise the negative effects and to make the experience as normal as possible. The process of choosing and eating food is not something we are conscious of, it doesn't take up a large part of our thinking and planning and neither should it for a patient. Using special tools such as straws is not normal and they draw attention to the person eating and so may be refused by patients even though the nurse thinks that it is a good idea; similarly some patients may use tools in their own home but not outside it. Patients should be able to completely depend on having the same choices offered to them as others would experience without having to ask for it. They should be able to say what and how they want to be fed, with what tools or devices and at what speed without feeling that they are being unreasonable. Once a meal begins they should be able to expect that their helper will stay with them throughout and give them their whole attention. Thus during meal times, the relationship between a patient and the person feeding them could be one of extraordinary closeness. The attention and care with which the nurse assists a patient to eat will directly affect the self-respect and level of control the patient experiences, thus affecting their sense of personhood. Martinsen et al. (2008, 2009) found that for the patients in their study, the meal was organised in order to increase the level of normality and reduce the levels of shame and embarrassment. The way it was done and the use of tools had to be weighed against these measures all the time.

There is an element of shame and embarrassment involved in being fed; not just in the receiving of help, but in the asking for it. Using tools and having food cut up could also be a source of shame and embarrassment, but not adapting risked being further embarrassed by having food dribbled down your chin or clothes. So some weighing up had to be done. As one respondent said, 'It is not humiliating for me to receive help with my meals. But it is humiliating to look like a pig' (Martinsen et al. 2008, p. 538). Helping someone to eat is an individually designed process, people who will permanently need help need to 'recognise themselves in every single feature' (Martinsen et al. 2008, p. 538) of the assisted eating process. This shows how the way we eat is so elementally bound up in personhood and how we recognise who we are.

When someone is cognitively impaired, for instance by dementia, personhood may be blurred but not absent, it is certainly vulnerable; the same amount of sensitive respect should be used. Consider this mealtime observed in a nursing home.

Nursing assistants typically approached residents without greeting them or verbally acknowledging what was about to happen. They usually stood next to residents while feeding them, rather than sitting and facing them. For many residents, this put the person feeding them out of their range of vision. Often nursing assistants conversed with each other while they fed the residents,... The effect was that staff members literally spoke over the residents heads.

(Ryvicker 2009, pp. 12–23)

Sometimes the mealtime is understandably seen as an opportunity for a sit down and a break by nurses or it's a chore which is best avoided. There is a challenge for nursing leaders in helping nurses to see feeding someone as a rewarding experience.

The spiritual care in helping someone to eat

Action	Spiritual rationale
• If you don't know the patient, introduce yourself, establish a relationship, make eye contact.	• Shows warmth, humanity and compassion.
• Find out as much as possible before hand about what the patients likes to eat and how. • Ask the patient what preferences they have in how they'd like to be helped. • Give as much choice as possible. Find out about any cultural and religious preferences. • Give your whole attention to the patient and don't allow yourself to be interrupted.	• Empowers the patient and shows that you value their opinion. • Demonstrates that you are at their service and are willing to be led by them.
• Talk to the person as you would with anyone while eating. Be sensitive to how much talk they want.	• Includes in the flow of life, values patient, shows care. Makes the patient feel cared for because you are interested in them.

• If you are wearing gloves, explain the infection control rationale. If there is no reason in policy, take them off.	• Shows solidarity and connection to the patient. To wear gloves makes the event a procedure. To not wear gloves makes it part of normal life.
• Respect the patient's wishes to eat alone or with others.	• Shows that you see them as an individual, able to make decisions and have preferences.
• Make eye contact and be wholly present.	• Shows respect and attention and empathy.

Conclusion

Food has connections with spirituality in many different ways. Decisions about what food to eat and how and where it is eaten express many aspects of our personality and culture. When these decisions are disturbed or denied it is easy to feel that our very identity is threatened and our place in our community is under attack. Nurses have to work hard to restore the patients' individuality and humanity against this assault. However, the effort is worth it because relieving anxiety and restoring wholeness and humanity in the area of eating and food will make a huge difference to the spiritual life and spiritual well-being of a patient.

Conclusion

Spiritual care has been written about and researched for 40 years, but up to now we haven't found a way to include spirituality into nursing in a way which is helpful to patients and which feels natural to nurses. The basis for this book is that this is not likely to happen until spirituality is incorporated into the everyday life of nurses. This means embedding spiritual care into relationships and into the physical personal care of nursing. The focus of most nursing care is the body and even mental health nurses who might instinctively shy from this idea will find a way to practice spiritual care through dealing with patients and clients as integrated physical and spiritual beings and not only as people with disordered minds. Nurses are in the privileged position of being able to touch and work with people's bodies in a unique way, yet they have been seduced into believing that talking was the only way to provide spiritual care. This book has challenged that view and argued that there is another way to provide spiritual care by embedding it into every encounter and relationship and into the physicality of everyday nursing and midwifery care.

Doctors, chaplains and psychiatrists have all assumed that the way nurses should provide spiritual care is little different from the way they do it. But they cannot rub a patient's back or soak a patient's feet. They are not there to hold a patients head when they are sick. They are not the ones to sit and hold the hand of someone in pain at 4 am. These other professionals are informed in a sentence in a consultation that someone is anxious, they never spend six hours at a stretch with patients so that they see and experience their anxiety, in the way that nurses do. They do not make the precious tea at midnight for the person who can't sleep. The nurse is the one who greets the woman coming for her mastectomy at the door of the ward, takes her from her family and explains how her day will be. The nurse is the only person allowed into a person's home with the sole purpose of helping them to wash; the midwife sits with the woman in labour, not arriving for any particular task, but simply to 'be with'.

This is the stuff of nurses' work and it is in these acts of care that that spiritual care in nursing unfolds.

It is time for nurses to find their own voice and explore the spirituality inherent in the *actual* work they do, not in a sanitised, ordered version of their day created by others.

This little book has barely touched on the ways in which nurses can give spiritual care. Hopefully my inadequate voice will inspire others to take this vision and to develop ever more creative ways to explore the true relationship between spirituality and nursing – not only to develop spiritual care, because that would be a very limited goal, but rather to use the concept of making all care spiritual to develop and improve everything that nurses do.

References

Age UK (2010) *Still Hungry to Be Heard* (London: Age UK).

Alavi, C. (1995) 'Breaking-in bodies: teaching, nursing, initiations or what's love got to do with it?' *Contemporary Nurse*, 18, 292–299.

Allan, H.T., Smith, P. (2009) 'How student nurses' supernumerary status affects the way they think about nursing', *Nursing Times*, 105(43), 10.

Appleton, C. (1993) 'The art of nursing: the experience of patients and nurses', *Journal of Advanced Nursing*, 18, 892–899.

Argyle, M. (1988) *Bodily Communication, 2nd ed.* (London: Methuen and Co.).

Åstedt-Kürki, P., Haggman-Laitila, A. (1992) 'Good nursing practice as perceived by clients: a starting point for the development of professional nursing', *Journal of Advanced Nursing*, 17, 1195–1199.

Autton, N. (1989) *Touch: An Exploration* (London: Darton, Longman, Todd).

Baldacchino, D. (2011) *Spiritual Care in a Hospital Setting: Conference paper*, Spiritual Care and Health Professions, 5th Bi-annual International Student Conference, Amsterdam.

Bates, J. (2007) 'In touch', *Nursing Standard*, 22(10), 25.

Batson, C.D., Schoenrade, P.A. (1991) 'Measuring religion as quest: (1) validity concerns', *Journal for the Scientific Study of Religion*, 30(4), 416–429.

Bottorff, J. (1991) 'The lived experience of being comforted by a nurse', *Phenomenology and Pedagogy*, 9, 237–252. Also online: Phenomenology Online. http://www.phenomenologyonline.com/sources/textorium/bottorff-joan-the-lived-experience-of-being-comforted-by-a-nurse/ (Accessed 15 December 2012).

Boughton, M. (1997) Embodied self, human biology and experience. In J. Lawler (ed.) *The Body in Nursing* (Melbourne, VIC: Churchill Livingstone), 155–175.

Bradshaw, A. (1997) 'Teaching spiritual care to nurses: an alternative approach', *International Journal of Palliative Nursing*, 3(1), 51–57.

Buber, M. (1970) *I and Thou*, Translated by Walter Kaufmann (New York: Charles Scribner's Son's).

Cameron, D. (2012) *Patients Not Paperwork*, Number 10: The Official Site of the British Prime Minister's Office. http://www.number10.gov.uk/news/patients-not-paperwork/ (Accessed 15 December 2012)

Campbell, A.V. (1984) *Moderated Love* (London: SPCK).

Care Quality Commission (2011) *Dignity and Nutrition for Older People: Review of Compliance* (London: CQC). http://www.cqc.org.uk/public/reports-surveys-and-reviews/themes-inspections/dignity-and-nutrition-older-people (Accessed 15 December 2012)

Cassell, E.J. (2004) *The Nature of Suffering and the Goals of Medicine, 2nd ed.* (Oxford: Oxford University Press).

Chang, A.M. (1995) 'Perceived functions and usefulness of health service support workers', *Journal of Advanced Nursing*, 21, 64–74.

Clark, C., Cross, J.R., Deane, D., Lowry, L.W. (1991) 'Spirituality: integral to quality care', *Holistic Nursing Practice*, 5(3), 67–76.

Clarke, J. (1997) *The Role of the Health Care Assistant in Direct Personal Care*, Unpublished Research, University College Worcester.

Clarke, J. (1999) 'The diminishing role of nurses in hands-on care', *Nursing Times*, 95(27), 48–49.

Clarke, J. (2006a) 'A discussion paper about "meaning" in the nursing literature on spirituality: an interpretation of meaning as "ultimate concern" using the work of Paul Tillich', *International Journal of Nursing Studies*, 43, 915–921.

Clarke, J. (2006b) 'Religion and spirituality: a discussion paper about negativity, reductionism and differentiation in nursing texts', *International Journal of Nursing Studies*, 43, 775–785.

Clarke, J. (2009) 'A critical view of how nursing has defined spirituality', *Journal of Clinical Nursing*, 18, 1666–1673.

Clarke, J. (2010) 'Body and soul in mental health care', *Mental Health, Religion and Culture*, 13(6), 649–657.

Clarke, J. (2011) Christianity and nursing. In M. Fowler, S. Riemer-Kirkham, R. Sawatzky, & E. Johnston Taylor (eds.) *Religion, Religious Ethics and Nursing* (New York: Springer).

Clebsch, W.A., Jaekle, C.R. (1975) *Pastoral Care in Historical Perspective* (New York: Aronson).

Clement, O. (1986) *On Human Being: A Spiritual Anthropology* (London: New City).

Climacus, J. (1982) *The Ladder of Divine Ascent: The Classics of Western Spirituality* (New York: Paulist Pres).

Comte-Sponville, A. (2007) *The Book of Atheist Spirituality* (London: Bantam Books).

Conco, D. (1995) 'Christian patients' views of spiritual care', *Western Journal of Nursing Research*, 17(3), 266–275.

Crawford, M.L. (1910) 'Why, when and how to bathe a fever patient', *The American Journal of Nursing*, 10(5), 314.

Csepregi, G. (2006) *The Clever Body* (Calgary, AB: Calgary University Press).

Culliford, L., Eagger, S. (2009) Assessing spiritual needs. In A. Powell & A. Sims (eds.) *Spirituality and Psychiatry* (London: The Royal College of Psychiatrists).

Davie, G. (1994) *Religion in Britain since 1945: Believing without Belonging* (Oxford: Blackwell).

Davie, G. (2007) Vicarious religion: a methodological challenge. In N.T. Ammerman (ed.) *Everyday Religion: Observing Modern Religious Lives* (New York: Oxford University Press), 21–37.

Davies, O. (2001) *A Theology of Compassion* (London: SCM Press).

De Hennezel, M. (1998) *Intimate Death: How the Dying Teach Us to Live* (London: Warner Books).

De Hennezel, M. (2011) *The Warmth of the Heart Prevents the Body from Rusting* (London: Pan Macmillan).

Department of Health (2009) *Religion or Belief: A Practical Guide for the NHS* (London: DH).

Dewar, B.J., Macleod-Clark, J. (1992) 'The role of the paid non-professional nursing helper: a review of the literature', *Journal of Advanced Nursing*, 17, 113–120.

Donahue, M.P. (1985) *Nursing: The Finest Art* (Missouri: C.V Mosby Co).

Donahue, M.J. (1985) 'Intrinsic and extrinsic religiousness': review and meta-analysis', *Journal of Personality and Social Psychology*, 48(2), 400–419.

Dougherty, L., Lister, S. (eds.) (2011) *The Royal Marsden Hospital Manual of Clinical Nursing Procedures, 8th ed.* (London: Wiley-Blackwell), 417–533.

Douglas, M. (2002) *Purity and Danger* (London: Routledge Classics).

Drew, N. (1986) 'Exclusion and confirmation: a phenomenology of patients' experiences with caregivers', *Image: Journal of Nursing Scholarship*, 18(2), 39–43.

Edvardsson, J.D., Sandman, P., Rasumssen, B. (2003) 'Meanings of giving touch in the care of older patients: becoming a valuable person and professional', *Journal of Clinical Nursing*, 12, 601–609.

Edwards, S. (1998) 'An anthropological interpretation of nurses' and patients' perceptions of the use of space and touch', *Journal of Advanced Nursing*, 28(4), 809–817.

Ellison, C.W. (1983) 'Spiritual well-being: conceptualisation and measurement', *Journal of Psychology and Theology*, 11(4), 330–340.

Estabrooks, C.A. (1987) 'Touch in nursing practice: a historical perspective', *Journal of Nursing History*, 2(2), 33–49.

Estabrooks, C., Morse, J.M. (1992) 'Towards a theory of touch: the touching process and acquiring a touching style', *Journal of Advanced Nursing*, 17, 448–456.

Falk-Rafael, A. (2001) 'Empowerment as a process of evolving consciousness: a model of empowered caring', *Advances in Nursing Science*, 24(1), 106.

Fenton, S. (2011) 'Reflections on lymphoedema, fungating wounds and the power of touch in the last weeks of life', *International Journal of Palliative Nursing*, 17(2), 60–66.

Field, T. (1999) 'American adolescents touch each other less and are more aggressive towards their peers as compared with French adolescents', *Adolescence*, 35(136), 753–758.

Firth-Cozens, J., Cornwell, J. (2009) *The Point of Care: Enabling Compassionate Care in Acute Hospital Settings* (London: Kings Fund).

Fosbinder, D. (1994) 'Patient perceptions of nursing care: an emerging theory of interpersonal competence', *Journal of Advanced Nursing*, 20(6), 1085–1093.

Fowler, M.D. (2009) 'Religion, bioethics and nursing practice', *Nursing Ethics*, 16(4), 393–404.

Fowler, M., Riemer-Kirkham, S., Sawatzky, R., Taylor, E.J. (eds.) (2011) *Religion, Religious Ethics and Nursing* (New York: Springer).

Frankl, V. (1984) *Man's Search for Meaning* (New York: Washington Square Press).

Fredriksson, L. (1999) 'Modes of relating in a caring conversation: a research synthesis on presence, touch and listening', *Journal of Advanced Nursing*, 30(5), 1167–1176.

Gadow, S.A. (1985) The nurse and patient: the caring relationship. In R. Bishop & J. Scudder (eds.) *Caring, Curing, Coping: Nurse, Physician, Patient Relationships* (Alabama: University of Alabama Press), 31–43.

Gastmans, C. (1998) 'Meals in nursing homes: an ethical appraisal', *Scandinavian Journal of Caring Science*, 12, 231–237.

Gee, P. (2006) *A Beginners Guide to Macmurray in a Philosophical Context*, The John Macmurray Fellowship Website: Further Reading. http://johnmacmurray.org/further-reading/a-beginners-guide-to-macmurray-in-a-philosophical-context/ (Accessed 24 January 2012).

Gleeson, M., Higgins, A. (2009) 'Touch in mental health nursing: an exploratory study of nurses views and perceptions', *Journal of Psychiatric and Mental Health Nursing*, 16, 382–389.

Goddard, N.C. (1995) 'Spirituality as integrative energy': a philosophical analysis as requisite precursor to holistic nursing practice', *Journal of Advanced Nursing*, 22, 808–815.

Goldberg, B. (1998) 'Connection: an exploration of spirituality in nursing care', *Journal of Advanced Nursing*, 27, 836–842.

Gordon, E.C. (1903) 'Some observations on the nursing of typhoid fever', *The American Journal of Nursing*, 3(8), 593–600.

Govier, I. (2000) 'Spiritual care in nursing: a systematic approach', *Nursing Standard*, 14(17), 32–36.

Grant, B.M., Giddings, L.S., Beale, J.E. (2005) 'Vulnerable bodies: competing discourse of intimate bodily care', *Journal of Nursing Education*, 44(11), 498–504.

Greasley, P., Chiu, L.F., Gartland, M. (2001) 'The concept of spiritual care in mental health nursing', *Journal of Advanced Nursing*, 33(5), 629–637.

Groenhout, R., Hotz, K., Joldersma, C. (2005) 'Embodiment, nursing practice, and religious faith: a perspective from one tradition', *Journal of Religion and Health*, 44(2), 147–160.

Guéguen, N., Vion, M. (2009) 'The effect of a practitioner's touch on a patient's medication compliance', *Psychology, Health & Medicine*, 14(6), 689–694.

Hardy, J. (2011) *Sometimes the Patient Just Wants a Hug*, Nursing Standard online. http://nursingstandard.rcnpublishing.co.uk/students/clinical-placements/patientcentred-care/building-bonds-with-patients/sometimes-the-patient-just-wants-a-hug/ (Accessed 15 December 2012).

Hay, D. (2000) 'Spirituality versus Individualism: why we should nurture relational consciousness', *International Journal of Children's Spirituality*, 5(1), 37–48.

Hay, D., Nye, R. (2006) *The Spirit of the Child, Revised ed.* (London: Jessica Kingsley).

Heelas, P., Woodhead, L. (2005) *The Spiritual Revolution: Why Religion Is Giving Way to Spirituality* (Oxford: Blackwell Publishing).

Hertenstein, M.J., Keltner, D., App, B., Bulleit, A., Jasolka, A.R. (2006) 'Touch communicates distinct emotions', *Emotion*, 6(3), 528–533.

Herth, K. (1993) 'Hope in the family caregiver of terminally ill people', *Journal of Advanced Nursing*, 18, 538–548

Howarth, G. (1998) '"Just live for today". Living, caring, ageing and dying', *Ageing and Society*, 18, 673–689.

Hungelmann, J., Kenkel-Rossi, E., Klassen, L., Stollenwerk, R. (1996) 'Focus on spiritual well-being: harmonious interconnectedness of mind-body-spirit. Use of the JAREL spiritual well-being scale', *Geriatric Nursing*, 17(6), 262–266.

Johnson, C. (2010) Dilemmas of spiritual assessment. In W. McSherry & L. Ross (eds.) *Spiritual Assessment in Healthcare Practice* (Keswick: M&K Publishing), 139–160.

Jourard, S.M. (1971) *The Transparent Self, Revised ed.* (New York: Van Nostrand)

Kaufmann, W. (1970) Prologue. In M. Buber (ed.) *I and Thou*, Translated by W. Kauffman (New York: Charles Scribner's Son's).

Kraus, R. (2009) 'The many faces of spirituality: a conceptual framework considering belly dance', *Implicit Religion*, 12, 51–72.

Lawler, J. (1991) *Behind the Screens: Nursing, Somology, and the Problem of the Body* (Melbourne, VIC: Churchill Livingstone) (Reissued 2006 by SUP).

Lear, M.W. (1980) *Heartsounds: The Story of Love and Loss* (New York: Simon and Schuster).

Leppanen-Montgomery, C. (1991) 'The care-giving relationship: paradoxical and transcendent aspects', *The Journal of Transpersonal Psychology*, 23(2), 91–104.

Levin, D.M. (1985) *The Body's Recollection of Being: Phenomenological Psychology and the Deconstruction of Nihilism* (London: Routledge and Kegan Paul).

Liehr, P.R. (1989) 'The core of true presence: a loving centre', *Nursing Science Quarterly*, 2(1), 7–8.

Louth, A. (1996) *Maximus the Confessor* (London: Routledge).

Lundman, B., Viglund, K., Aléx, L., Jonsén, E., Norberg, A., Fischer, A.S., Strandberg, G., Nygren, B. (2011) 'Development and psychometric properties of the Inner Strength Scale, *International Journal of Nursing Studies*, 48, 1266–1274.

Macleod, M. (1994) 'It's the little things that count: the hidden complexity of everyday clinical practice', *Journal of Clinical Nursing*, 3(6), 361–368.

Macmurray, J. (1995) *Search for Reality in Religion* (London: Quaker Home Service & the John Macmurray Society).

Malinski, V.M. (2002) 'Developing a nursing perspective on spirituality and healing', *Nursing Science Quarterly*, 15, 281–287.

Marcel, G. (1969) *The Philosophy of Existence*, Translated by M. Harari (Freeport, NY: Books for Libraries Press).

Marcus Aurelius (2005), *Meditations*, Translated by George Long (Stilwell: Digireads).

Martinsen, B., Harder, I., Biering-Sorensen, F. (2008) 'The meaning of assisted feeding for people living with spinal cord injury: a phenomenological study', *Journal of Advanced Nursing*, 62(5), 533–540.

Martinsen, B., Harder, I., Biering-Sorensen, F. (2009) 'Sensitive cooperation: a basis for assisted feeding', *Journal of Clinical Nursing*, 18, 708–715.

Martsolf, D.S., Mickley, J.R. (1998) 'The concept of spirituality in nursing theories: differing world-views and extent of focus', *Journal of Advanced Nursing*, 27, 294–303.

McCabe, C., Timmins, F. (2006) *Communication Skills for Nursing Practice* (Basingstoke: Palgrave Macmillan).

McGuire, M.B. (1990) 'Religion and the body: rematerializing the human body in social sciences of religion', *Journal for the Scientific Study of Religion*, 29(3), 283–296.

McGuire, M.B. (2007) Embodied practices: negotiation and resistance. In N.T. Ammerman (ed.) *Everyday Religion: Observing Modern Lives* (Oxford: Oxford University Press), 187–200.

McIntosh, M.A. (1998) *Mystical Theology* (Oxford: Blackwell).

McKenzie, R. (2002) Philosophical congruence for use of the self. In D. Freshwater (ed.) *Therapeutic Nursing* (London: Sage), 22–38.

McMahon, R., Pearson, A. (1998) *Nursing as Therapy, 2nd ed.* (Cheltenham: Stanley Thornes).

McSherry, W. (2006) *Making Sense of Spirituality in Nursing and Health Care, 2nd ed.* (London: Jessica Kingsley).

McSherry, W. (2010) Spiritual assessment: definition, categorisation and features. In W. McSherry & L. Ross (eds.) *Spiritual Assessment in Healthcare Practice* (Keswick: M&K Publishing), 57–78.

McSherry, W., Draper, P. (1998) 'The debates emerging from the literature surrounding the concept of spirituality as applied to nursing', *Journal of Advanced Nursing*, 27, 683–691.

McSherry, W., Jamieson, S. (2011) 'An online survey of nurses' perceptions of spirituality and spiritual care', *Journal of Clinical Nursing*, 20(11/12), 1757–1767.

McSherry, W., Ross, L. (eds.) (2010) *Spiritual Assessment in Healthcare Practice* (Keswick: M&K Publishing).

Melia, K.M. (1983) 'Doing nursing and being professional', *Nursing Times*, 79(22), 28–30.

Merleau-Ponty, M. (1962) *The Phenomenology of Perception* (London: Routledge & Kegan Paul).

Miller, W. (1997) *The Anatomy of Disgust* (Boston, MA: Harvard University Press).

Miner-Williams, D. (2007) 'Connectedness in the nurse-patient relationship: a grounded theory study', *Issues in Mental Health Nursing*, 28, 1215–1234.

Mitchell S., Roberts, P. (2009) Psychosis. In C. Cook, A. Powell, & A. Sims (eds.) *Spirituality and Psychiatry* (London: RCPsych Publications), 39–61.

Moriarty, M. (2011) 'A conceptualisation of children's spirituality arising out of recent research', *International Journal of Children's Spirituality*, 16(3), 271–285.

Morse, J.M., Bottorff, J., Anderson, G., O'Brien, B., Solberg, S. (1992) 'Beyond empathy: expanding expressions of caring', *Journal of Advanced Nursing*, 17, 809–821.

Morse, J.M., Bottorff, J.L., Hutchinson, S. (1995) 'The paradox of comfort', *Nursing Research*, 44(1), 14–19.

Moss, B., Clarke, J., Moody, I. (2011) Educating for spiritual care. In P. Gilbert (ed.) *Spirituality and Mental Health* (Brighton: Pavilion), 281–297.

Mother Thekla (1997) *Eternity Now: An Introduction to Orthodox Spirituality* (Norwich: The Canterbury Press).

Narayanasamy, A., Clissett, P., Parumal, L., Thompson, D., Annasamy, S., Edge, R. (2004) 'Responses to the spiritual needs of older people', *Journal of Advanced Nursing*, 48(1), 6–16.

Narayanasamy, A., Narayanasamy, M. (2008) 'The healing power of prayer and its implications for nursing', *British Journal of Nursing*, 17(6), 394–398.

Nathan, B. (2007) 'The sense of touch – a philosophical surprise', *Journal of Holistic Healthcare*, 4(4), 24–31.

National Institute for Health and Clinical Excellence (2004) *Improving Supportive and Palliative Care for Adults with Cancer*. www.nice .org.uk/nicemedia/live/10893/28816/28816.pdf (accessed 22 January 2011).

National Patient Safety Agency (2007) *Protected Mealtimes Review: Findings and Recommendations Report* (London: NPSA).

Nettleton, S. (1995) *The Sociology of Health and Illness* (Cambridge: Polity Press).

Newitt, M. (2010) 'The role and skills of a hospital chaplain: reflections based on a case study', *Practical Theology*, 3(2), 163–177.

NHS Education for Scotland (2009) *Spiritual Care Matters: An Introductory Resource for All NHS Scotland Staff* (Edinburgh: NES).

Noble, A., Jones, C. (2010) 'Getting it right: oncology nurses' understanding of spirituality', *International Journal of Palliative Nursing*, 16(11), 565–569.

Nolan, S. (2011) 'Psychospiritual care: new concept for old content – towards a new paradigm for non-religious spiritual care', *Journal for the Study of Spirituality*, 1(1), 50–64.

North American Nursing Diagnosis Association (NANDA) (2012) *Nursing Diagnoses: Definitions and Classification 2012–14, 9th ed.* (Chichester: Wiley Blackwell).

Nursing and Midwifery Council (2008) *The Code: Standards of Conduct, Performance and Ethics for Nurses and Midwives* (London: NMC).

Nursing and Midwifery Council (2009) *Standards for Pre-registration Midwifery Education* (London: NMC).

Nursing and Midwifery Council (2010) *Standards for Pre-registration Nursing Education: Essential Skill Clusters* (London: NMC).

Nygren, B., Norberg, A., Lundman, B. (2007) 'Inner strength as disclosed in narratives of the oldest old', *Qualitative Health Research*, 17(8), 1060–1073.

Office of National Statistics (2011) 'Religion in England and Wales'. http://www.ons.gov.uk/ons/rel/census/2011-census/key-statistics-for-local-authorities-in-england-and-wales/rpt-religion.html (Accessed 20 January 2013).

Öhman, M., Söderberg, S., Lundman, B. (2003) 'Hovering between suffering and enduring: the meaning of living with serious chronic illness', *Qualitative Health Research*, 13, 528–542.

O'Lynn, C., Krautscheid, L. (2011) 'How should I touch you': a qualitative study of attitudes on intimate touch in nursing, *American Journal of Nursing*, 111(3), 24–31.

Orsi, R.A. (2005) *Between Heaven and Earth: The Religious Worlds People Make and the Scholars Who Study Them* (Princeton, NJ: Princeton University Press).

Palamas, G. (1983) *Triads: The Classics of Western Spirituality* (Mahwah, NJ: Paulist Press).

Pargament, K.I. (1997) *The Psychology of Religion and Coping* (New York: The Guilford Press).

Parkes, M., Gilbert, P. (2011) 'Professional's calling: mental healthcare staff's attitudes to spiritual care', *Implicit Religion*, 14(1), 23–43.

Patterson, C. (2011a) 'Nasty Nurses? Tell me something new', *The Independent*, 16th February. http://www.independent.co.uk/opinion/commentators/christina-patterson/christina-patterson-nasty-nurses-tell-me-something-new-2215918.html (Accessed 15 December 2012)

Patterson, C (2011b) 'Care to be a Nurse', *Four Thought, Radio 4*, 15th July. http://www.bbc.co.uk/programmes/b010mrzt

Pattison, S. (2010) 'Spirituality and spiritual care made simple: a suggestive, normative and essentialist approach', *Practical Theology*, 3(3), 351–366.

Pearce, E. (1969) *Nurse and Patient: Human Relations in Nursing, 3rd ed.* (London: Faber and Faber).

Perry, L. (2008) 'Assisted feeding', *Journal of Advanced Nursing*, 63(5), 511.

Perry, L., McLaren, S. (2003) 'Coping and adaptation at six months after stroke: experiences with eating disabilities', *International Journal of Nursing Studies*, 40, 185–195.

Picco, E., Santoro, R., Garrino, L. (2010) 'Dealing with the patient's body in nursing: nurse's ambiguous experience in clinical practice', *Nursing Inquiry*, 17(1), 38–45.

Piles, C.L. (1990) 'Providing spiritual care', *Nurse Educator*, 15(1), 36–41.

Pollard, T. (2009) 'The place of religion in nursing practice', *British Journal of Nursing*, 18(4), 217.

Post-White, J., Ceronsky, C., Kreitzer, M.J., Nickelson, K., Drew, D., Mackey, K.W., Koopmeiners, L., Gutnecht, S. (1996) 'Hope, spirituality, sense of coherence and quality of life in patients with cancer', *Oncology Nursing Forum*, 23(10), 1571–1579.

Price, R. (1995) *A Whole New Life: An Illness and a Healing* (London: Plume Penguin).

Pridmore, P., Pridmore, J. (2004) 'Promoting the spiritual development of sick children', *International Journal of Children's Spirituality*, 9(1), 21–38.

Prothero, S. (2011) *God Is Not One: The Eight Rival Religions That Run the World and Why Their Differences Matter* (New York: Harper Collins).

Puchalski, C. (2010) The spiritual history: an essential element of patient-centred care. In W. McSherry & L. Ross (eds.) *Spiritual Assessment in Healthcare Practice* (Keswick: M&K Publishing), 79–95.

Reimer, H.D., Keller, H.H. (2009) 'Mealtimes in nursing homes: striving for person centred care', *Journal of Nutrition for the Elderly*, 28, 327–347.

Romero, J.H. (2000) 'Comprehensive versus holistic care: case studies of chronic disease', *Journal of Holistic Nursing*, 18(4), 352–361.

Roper, N. (2002) Interview at RCN Congress, *The Answer*, Autumn (London: RCN).

Routasalo, P., Isola, A. (1996) 'The right to touch and be touched', *Nursing Ethics*, 3(2), 165–175.

Royal College of Nursing (2003) *Defining Nursing* (London: RCN).

Royal College of Psychiatrists (2011) *Recommendations for Psychiatrists on Spirituality and Religion: Position Statement* (London: Royal College of Psychiatrists).

Ryvicker, M. (2009) 'Preservation of self in the nursing home: contradictory practices within two models of care', *Journal of Aging Studies*, 23, 12–23.

Scheper-Hughes, M., Lock, M.M. (1987) 'The mindful body: a prolegomenon to future work in medical anthropology', *Medical Anthropology Quarterly*, 1(1), 6–41.

Schmemann, A. (1987) *The Eucharist* (New York: St Vladimir's Seminary Press).

Schneiders, S.M. (1989) 'Spirituality in the academy', *Theological Studies*, 50, 676–697.

Shaver, W.A. (2002) 'Suffering and the role of abandonment of self', *Journal of Hospice and Palliative Nursing*, 4(1), 46–53.

Sheldrake, P. (2007) *A Brief History of Spirituality* (Oxford: Blackwell).

Short, P. (1997) Picturing the body in nursing. In J. Lawler (ed.) *The Body in Nursing* (Melbourne, VIC: Churchill Livingstone), 7–11.

Sims, A., Cook, C. (2009) Spirituality in psychiatry. In C. Cook, A. Powell, & A. Sims (eds.) *Spirituality and Psychiatry* (London: The Royal College of Psychiatrists), 1–16.

Smith, P., McSherry, W. (2004) 'Spirituality and child development: a concept analysis', *Journal of Advanced Nursing*, 45(3), 307–315.

Smuts, J. (1927) *Holism and Evolution* (London: Macmillan).

Smyth, T., Allen, S. (2011) 'Nurses' experiences assessing the spirituality of terminally ill patients in acute clinical practice', *International Journal of Palliative Nursing*, 17(7), 337–343.

Speck, P. (2005) 'The evidence base for spiritual care', *Nursing Management*, 12(6), 28–31.

Stark, R. (1999) 'Secularisation, R.I.P', *Sociology of Religion*, 60(3), 249–273.

Starr, S.S. (2008) 'Authenticity: a concept analysis', *Nursing Forum*, 43(2), 55–62.

Stein, M. (2008) *The Lonely Patient: How We Experience Illness* (New York: Harper Perennial).

Stern, J. (2001) 'John Macmurray, spirituality, community and real schools', *International Journal of Children's Spirituality*, 6(1), 25–39.

Stern, L.J., James, S. (2006) 'Every person matters: enabling spirituality education for nurses', *Journal of Clinical Nursing*, 15, 897–704.

Swinton, J. (2001) *Spirituality and Mental Health Care: Rediscovering a 'Forgotten' Dimension* (London: Jessica Kingsley).

Swinton, J., Pattison, S. (2010) 'Moving beyond clarity: towards a thin, vague, and useful understanding of spirituality in nursing care', *Nursing Philosophy*, 11, 226–237.

Tacey, D. (2003) *The Spirituality Revolution: The Emergence of Contemporary Spirituality* (Sydney: Harper Collins).

Tanyi, R. (2002) 'Towards a clarification of the meaning of spirituality', *Journal of Advanced Nursing*, 39(5), 500–509.

Tanyi, R.A., Stehle-Werner, J., Gentry-Recine, A.C., Sperstad, R.A. (2006) 'Perceptions of incorporating spirituality into their care: a phenomenological study of female patients on hemodyalisis', *Nephrology Nursing Journal*, 33(5), 532–538.

Taylor, B. (1992) 'From helper to human: a reconceptualization of the nurse as a person', *Journal of Advanced Nursing*, 19(9), 1042–1049.

Taylor, B. (1994) *Being Human: Ordinariness in Nursing* (Melbourne, VIC: Churchill Livingstone).

Taylor, B. (1995) 'Nursing as healing work', *Contemporary Nurse*, 4(3), 100–106.

Taylor, E.J. (2011) Religion and patient care. In M.D. Fowler et al. (eds.) *Religion, Religious Ethics and Nursing* (New York: Springer), 313–338.

Taylor, E.J, Mamier, I. (2005) 'Spiritual care nursing: what cancer patients and family caregivers want', *Journal of Advanced Nursing*, 49(3), 260–267.

Tear Fund (2007) *Churchgoing in the UK* (London: Tearfund).

The Patients Association (2011) *We've Been Listening, Have You Been Learning?* (Middlesex: The Patients Association). http://patients-association.com/default.aspx?tabid= 80&Id= 23 (Accessed 15 December 2012)

Thunberg, L. (1995) *Microcosm and Mediator: The Theological Anthropology of Maximus the Confessor, 2nd ed.* (Illinois: Open Court Publishing).

Tschudin, V. (1999) *Nurses Matter: Reclaiming Our Professional Identity* (London: Macmillan).

Turner, B.S. (1991) *Religion and Social Theory, 2nd ed.* (London: Sage).

Tutton, E. (1998) An exploration of touch and its use in nursing. In R. McMahon & A. Pearson (eds.) *Nursing as Therapy, 2nd ed.* (Cheltenham: Stanley-Thornes), 168–200.

Twigg, J. (2000) *Bathing: The Body in Community Care* (London: Routledge).

van den Berg, J. (1955) *The Phenomenological Approach to Psychiatry* (Springfield, IL: Thomas).

van Hooft, S. (2002) Towards a philosophy of caring and spirituality for a secular age. In B. Rumbold (ed.) *Spirituality and Palliative Care* (Oxford: Oxford University Press), 38–51

van Hooft, S. (2006) *Caring about Health* (Aldershot: Ashgate Publishing).

van Manen, M. (1998) 'Modalities of body experience in illness and health', *Qualitative Health Research*, 8(1), 7–24.

van Manen, M. (1999) The pathic nature of enquiry and nursing. In I. Madjar & J. Walton (eds.) *Nursing and the Experience of Illness: Phenomenology in Practice* (London: Routledge), 17–35.

van Manen, M. (2007) *Researching Lived Experience* (Ontario: The Althouse Press).

Van Ness, P.H. (ed.) (1996) *Spirituality and the Secular Quest* (London: SCM Press).

von Essen, L., Sjödén, P. (1991) 'Patient and staff perceptions of caring: review and replication', *Journal of Advanced Nursing*, 16, 1363–1374.

Walter, T. (1985) *All You Love is Need* (London: SPCK).

Walter, T. (1997) 'The ideology and organisation of spiritual care: three approaches', *Palliative Medicine*, 11, 21–30.

Watson, M., Lucas, C., Hoy, A., Wells, J. (2009) *Oxford Handbook of Palliative Care* (Oxford: Oxford University Press).

Ware, K. (1995) *The Orthodox Way, Revised ed.* (New York: St Vladimir's Seminary Press).

Ware, K. (2002) *The Unity of the Human Person: The Body-Soul Relationship in Orthodox Theology*, Proceedings of the Congress of Sciences, Technologies and Orthodoxy, Athens. Myriobiblos Website. http://www.myriobiblos.gr/texts/english/wear_unity_1.html (Accessed 23 February 2012).

Whitaker, A. (2010) 'The body as existential midpoint – the aging and dying body of nursing home residents', *Journal of Aging Studies*, 24, 96–104.

Williams, R. (1998) 'Lear and Eurydice: religious experience, crisis and change', *Spirituality and Religious Experience, The Way Supplement*, 92, 75–84.

Woods, M. (2011) Patient comfort. In L. Dougherty & S. Lister (eds.) *The Royal Marsden Hospital Manual of Clinical Nursing Procedures, 8th ed.* (London: Wiley-Blackwell), 417–533.

Wysong, P.R., Driver, E. (2009) 'Patients' perceptions of nurses' skill', *Critical Care Nurse*, 29, 24–37.

Zinnbauer, B.J., Pargament, K.I., Scott, A.B. (1999) 'The emerging meanings of religiousness and spirituality: problems and prospects', *Journal of Personality*, 67(6), 889–919.

Index